2

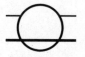

RESEARCHING DISABILITY ISSUES

Disability, Human Rights and Society
Series Editor: Professor Len Barton, University of Sheffield

The *Disability, Human Rights and Society* series reflects a commitment to a particular view of 'disability' and a desire to make this view accessible to a wider audience. The series approach defines 'disability' as a form of oppression and identifies the ways in which disabled people are marginalized, restricted and experience discrimination. The fundamental issue is not one of an individual's inabilities or limitations, but rather a hostile and unadaptive society.

Authors in this series are united in the belief that the question of disability must be set within an equal opportunities framework. The series gives priority to the examination and critique of those factors that are unacceptable, offensive and in need of change. It also recognizes that any attempt to redirect resources in order to provide opportunities for discriminated people cannot pretend to be apolitical. Finally, it raises the urgent task of establishing links with other marginalized groups in an attempt to engage in a common struggle. The issue of disability needs to be given equal significance to those of race, gender and age in equal opportunities policies. This series provides support for such a task.

Anyone interested in contributing to the series is invited to approach the Series Editor at the Division of Education, University of Sheffield.

Current and forthcoming titles

M. Corker: *Deaf and Disabled, or Deafness Disabled?*
M. Moore, S. Beazley and J. Maelzer: *Researching Disability Issues*
A. Roulstone: *Enabling Technology: Disabled People, Work and New Technology*
C. Thomas: *Female Forms: Disabled Women in Social Context*
A. Vlachou: *Struggles for Inclusive Education: An Ethnographic Study*

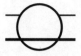

RESEARCHING DISABILITY ISSUES

Michele Moore
Sarah Beazley
June Maelzer

Open University Press
Buckingham · Philadelphia

Open University Press
Celtic Court
22 Ballmoor
Buckingham
MK18 1XW

and
1900 Frost Road, Suite 101
Bristol, PA 19007, USA

First Published 1998

A catalogue record of this book is available from the British Library

ISBN 0 335 19803 1 (pb)   0 335 19804 X (hb)

Library of Congress Cataloging-in-Publication Data
Moore, Michele.
   Researching disability issues / Michele Moore, Sarah Beazley, June Maelzer.
      p.   cm. – (Disability, human rights and society)
   Includes bibliographical references and index.
   ISBN 0-335-19804-X (hbk) – ISBN 0-335-19803-1 (pbk)
   1. Sociology of disability–Research.   2. Handicapped–Research.   I. Beazley,
Sarah.   II. Maelzer, June, 1942–   .   III. Title.   IV. Series.
HV1568.M66   1997
362.4'07'2–dc21   97-23228
                                                                                         CIP

Typeset by Type Study, Scarborough
Printed in Great Britain by St Edmundsbury Press Ltd, Bury St Edmunds, Suffolk

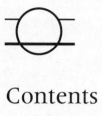

Contents

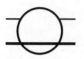

Series editor's preface

The Disability, Human Rights and Society series reflects a commitment to a social model of disability and a desire to make this view accessible to a wide audience. 'Disability' is viewed as a form of oppression and the fundamental issue is not one of an individual's inabilities or limitations, but rather a hostile and unadaptive society.

Priority is given to identifying and challenging those barriers to change, including the urgent task of establishing links with other marginalized groups and thus seeking to make connections between class, gender, race, age and disability factors.

The series aims to further establish disability as a serious topic of study, one in which the latest research findings and ideas can be seriously engaged with.

This book is a refreshingly open, readable and highly reflective account of research practices from insider perspectives. It is a very important contribution to the increasing attempts by researchers committed to a social model of disability, to develop a more enabling research practice.

The authors have focused on their own research activities in order to highlight some of the disabling aspects of research. In a vividly illustrative way they have effectively captured some of the key issues including questions of power, rights, commitment, interpersonal dynamics and moving the personal to the political, as they relate to the relationships between researchers and disabled people.

Developing a critical, rights-based approach to disability research is an extremely demanding task involving the researcher in a serious critical engagement of their values, presuppositions and practices. Fundamental questions need to be engaged with, including: What is the purpose of research? Who is to benefit from it? In what ways is research oppressive? When, how and with what consequence should disabled people participate in the research process? For the authors of this book, such questions are intended to challenge traditional conceptions of the role of the researcher and to place disabled people at the centre of disability research.

Research is often a lonely activity and one in which the actual process of the research act is hidden and shrouded in mystery. Part of the struggle to make research more relevant and challenging, is to demystify the social relations of the research process. The authors of this book provide a significant contribution towards achieving this goal, by highlighting the shifting patterns in their own thinking and encouraging other researchers to do the same. The authors provide 'thinking points' which are intended to foster such a disposition in the reader.

This form of research agenda is a demanding and disturbing task. The authors clearly demonstrate that both the thinking and working involved in the production of this book has been a very uncomfortable process. Even towards the end of the book, the tensions and difficulties are exemplified in the position of and relationships with the disabled co-author. Learning in terms of listening to one another, earning each other's respect and supporting one another leaves no room for complacency or arrogance.

This book is essential reading for all those who are concerned to work towards the establishment of a form of thinking and research in which disabled people have a significant role to play.

Professor Len Barton
Sheffield

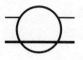

Acknowledgements

Many people have provided inspiration and encouragement for this book. In particular we would like to thank all those individual disabled people and their families who have contributed their experiences and views to our projects. Many disabled writers have been instrumental in shaping our thinking, but none more so than Mike Oliver, who nurtured both the original project, and ensuing reflections which turned out to be the stimulus for this book. We also want to thank Len Barton, for his time, commitment and most helpful contribution to the development of our ideas in his role as series editor, though of course we acknowledge, as is usual in these remarks, that any final shortcomings are entirely our own. Last but not least, we must thank our families and friends for encouragement and for a *great* deal of support in our writing of this book.

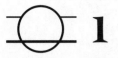 1

Questions and commitments in disability research

What this book is about

This book is an attempt to further the development of a critical approach to research in the field of disability studies and is intended to meet a need among researchers, including students, for rigorous reflection on inquiries concerning disabled people's lives. Disability research has been in a state of transformation and transition since 1992 when disabled researchers and their non-disabled peers set out to radically alter the basis of disability research production (Oliver 1992). Since then, many writers have exposed and debated the dilemmas and complexities facing those researching disability issues (Barnes 1992; Oliver 1992; Rioux and Bach 1994; Clough and Barton 1995; T. Shakespeare 1996). This book aims to complement these writings by providing a source of authentic examples of applied research which has sought to respond to the challenge of developing a new critical paradigm for disability research. This means that the book is more about processes than products. Chapters examine real projects with a view to illuminating the range of preoccupations with which disability researchers are routinely confronted.

We hope that this book will act as a marker in the development of enabling critical disability inquiry; the research reported is itself part of the problem we are commenting on, but will possibly suggest new positions and provide meaningful stimulus for those operating in the field. Throughout the text we try to make problematic research practice visible and to call for agitation and resistance where relations between the researcher and those being researched serve to marginalize the input of disabled people in the process of research and attendant production of knowledge. Focal material is intended to provide thought-provoking and topical insights into disability research, and wherever possible to illuminate human rights and society issues.

Starting points

We start from the position that as far as many disabled people are concerned, most disability research is a waste of time (Oliver 1992). Major investigations of disability matters can be critically reviewed in terms of their prospects for promoting disabled people's rights and found to undermine the promotion of disabled people's own agendas (Abberley 1992; Hirst and Baldwin 1994; Gregory *et al*. 1996). Consequently we began thinking about ways in which some of the research projects we have conducted – in different positions, for example as postgraduate students, practitioners or academic researchers, and as a trio of disabled and non-disabled women – tell several stories, produce multiple outcomes and are open to a variety of interpretations. A stringent look back has expanded our understanding of how disability research can function to reproduce disadvantage, inequality and disablement. Perhaps, by bringing the difficulties of our work into view, we can begin to unveil opportunities through which to further the process of more enabling disability research production.

An important motivation behind the book is to press readers to consider the politics underlying disability research projects. We give a comprehensive overview of what went on in some of our own work, in order to supplement and amplify theoretical understandings of how research could be, through a critical look at how research often actually is. Writing the book has necessarily entailed a thorough re-examination of ourselves as researchers, and demanded a close look at how our projects and other writings reflect the search for a critical disability research formula, one in which the promotion of disabled people's own priorities is uppermost.

Our interpretations frequently promote rejection of conventional criteria set for researchers in the human and social sciences. In arriving at this contention we have had to greatly extend our view of useful research practice. Thus we critically consider the different starting points of each project reported, examine research construction, and review the extent to which the completed work fits, or conversely does not fit, with our current thinking and ways of working. As a chronicle of research which should have been done differently, the book is at times depressing and threatens to overwhelm the everyday researcher but our aim is to acknowledge difficulties and in so doing, to untangle more promising avenues for future disability research.

As a starting point in any research, the theoretical model which underpins a project is always at issue. The language and discourse of disability research often shows investigators to be operating from *medical* and *individual* models of disability in which disability is seen as intrinsically related to a person's impairment. Within these approaches, the experience of disability is seen to stem from the individual, and consequently an individual-blaming philosophy informs research design. More dangerously, however, as all self-respecting researchers know, research design moulds research findings. Any research which is based on an individual model of disability will inevitably recycle individual-blaming images of disabled people and consequently inform relevant practical and policy issues in highly inauspicious ways. Such research is invariably oppressive and sweeps aside the generic and collective interests of disabled people (Rioux and Bach 1994; Clough and Barton 1995; Oliver 1996). It is not then surprising to find that many disabled people have called for a rejection of research based on individual and oppressive models of disability (Oliver 1990, 1992; Abberley 1992; Morris 1992b; Oliver 1996; Barnes 1997).

Within our own research endeavours we start with the view that disability is socially constructed and that explanations for disablement are to be found within the context of a person's life, rather than within individuals themselves. Our own disability research projects are now operationalized within this paradigm, but we also reflect on the implications of restricted engagement with the social model in some of our earlier studies. We now feel that *only* a critical approach to disability research, rooted firmly in social model discourse and practice, enables a human rights perspective to be given to issues which shape disabled people's lives. It is only with this approach that research can explore the extent to which fundamental rights, such as equal access to equal opportunities and to full inclusion in society, are recognized and promoted in the face of prejudice and excluding practices. Research which is structured in relation to the social model of disability is not 'disabled people blaming' but calls a disabling society to account. It is these ideas that form the basis of this book.

These arguments can be traced back to the suggestion put forward by Oliver (1992) that what is needed is 'emancipatory' disability research, which is carried out by disabled people and aimed at challenging routine oppression in their daily lives. Morris (1992a) has argued that disability research should also play a role in facilitating personal liberation of disabled people. Researchers are called upon to make their research skills and methodological expertise available to disabled people to use in pursuit of their own aspirations and concerns. En route towards the attainment of emancipatory ways of doing disability research, Zarb (1992) envisages a form of 'participatory research' which seeks to optimize partnership between researchers and disabled people. Research which aspires to be participatory and/or emancipatory has to be characterized by rigorous evaluation of questions of control. Who decides what the research will be about, how it will be conducted, and how far disabled people are engaged in central decision-making processes about a project and its outcomes, are all critical determinants of participation and hence of emancipatory prospects.

As French (1988) has indicated, academic mystique surrounding research has led to the exclusion of many people, disabled and non-disabled, from the research process and this is something we feel strongly is a barrier in need of dismantling. Mystification of research objectives and techniques has, in the past, led to a neglect of personal experience in investigations of disability, encouraged projects which are irrelevant to those who are being researched and recycled oppression and exploitation through fragmenting knowledge and reproducing marginalization of disability issues. These are all problems which we have tried, in various ways and with varying degrees of (limited) success, to resist in our own research work. What we note, based on our experience, is that stubborn structural, ideological and institutional barriers surround a researcher's efforts and these cannot be effortlessly thought away. We hope to illustrate challenges that everyday researchers come up against in trying to develop a critical and emancipatory disability research approach which is fully mindful of human rights issues. Being critical about self in terms of values, presuppositions and practices is an essential part of developing a critical disability research process, particularly when reflections can be made in association with others and in relation to the voices of disabled people.

We are not aiming to construct a particular image of what disability research should be in this book, but to tease out implications of a variety of situations in which researchers can find themselves through looking back at personal experience. We take a self-conscious look at scope for criticality in our own work. It may appear as if we had remarkable clarity at the time, which is, of course, not so. It has become possible to see points at which well-intentioned research switched to being potentially abusive, or points at which our own responses became subversive, only in retrospect. Often our individual efforts to resist pressures shaping a project were futile at the time, but they may suggest ideas for more effective collective resistance. It very quickly becomes clear that other than the need for critical reflection, and for unswerving commitment to making human rights issues explicit, we cannot pin-point what the essential ingredients of good disability research are, and the range of experience which the book analyses provides insight into why this might be so.

We can, however, begin to say from experience what good disability research is *not* like. We agree with Stone and Priestley (1996) and Oliver (1997) that certain core principles must characterize critical disability research. For us, it should not be embedded in, or regulated by, medical model ideologies; it should not attempt to be neutral or to disregard the impact of oppression on disabled people's lives; it should not reproduce the familiar, and so leave disabling personal, political or practical barriers unchallenged; it should not exclude disabled people from its process or productions; it should not be controlled entirely by non-disabled people and it should not be reluctant to venture in to unmapped theoretical and methodological territory. These are, at least, some of our personally agreed starting points.

We hope that the book will be used as a resource which may stimulate readers to reflect on their own assumptions and on practices that play a part in the conduct of their own disability research. To assist with this, we have included 'Thinking Points' linked to each chapter. A range of different strategies are suggested in these sections: pointers to important issues that have emerged in the chapter, questions that require readers to ponder and reconceptualize if they are willing so to do; and tasks that encourage readers to implement change and create new alliances. The purpose of this book is not only to identify ways in which our own research has been responsible for oppressions and inequities, but also to engage researchers with the task of bringing about change in their own.

Our position as researchers

We came together as a group of three women with expertise in different areas but a shared interest in disability. The research contexts we have selected reflect our research and professional interests (two as psychologists and one as a speech and language therapist) as well as our experience of disability (one of us as a disabled person and all of us with experience of disability within our own families). We are writing as academics trained in the conventional way, to be firmly attached to the fantasy of collecting 'objective' data, who have had to face the considerable personal cost of deconstructing our original research understandings in order to pursue meaningful research in the field of disability studies.

Finding a way of dealing with the necessary reconceptualization of what research is about has at times turned out to be a major debilitating factor in our careers. For instance, pursuit of a radical framework for inquiry has often placed our ideas at odds with the criteria for projects adopted by conventional research sponsors. Similarly, within universities where our research projects are located, criteria for scholarship are laid down by the Higher Education Funding Council's (HEFC) Research Assessment Exercise and used to monitor and evaluate an individual's professional performance, but our research activities largely evade these. This is because to attract merit in HEFC terms, research has typically – although not necessarily in all cases – been required to employ design, methodologies and representations which, in our view, subscribe to the oppression of disabled people (T. Shakespeare 1996). In order, for example, to uncover the realities of disabled people's lives, we believe subjectivity needs to be celebrated and so a partisan philosophy is an intrinsic part of our approach. However, such a view, being at odds with a long tradition of positivism in science, is hard to advocate within the parameters of HEFC evaluation procedures since research which fits with the existing state of things tends to be most highly approved. Similarly, HEFC assessment criteria specify that research publications which will be held in greatest esteem are those which appear 'in publications with rigorous editorial and refereeing standards' (Higher Education Funding Council 1996), but for our purposes, such outputs are most unlikely to get noticed by non-academic disabled people.

Consequently, an important question for us has been 'who do we want to value our research?' We have concluded that the audience of disabled people matters more to us than the erstwhile bodies which approve, control and evaluate research activity within conventional academic life. This has not been easy to accept. Much of our work is insufficiently rarefied – in the sense of being suitable for publication in refereed academic journals – to gain recognition, because we have remained determined to maximize relevance to disabled people's own aspirations and thus to present ideas differently. This issue, of who values the research, will be returned to throughout the book; it is critical even when researchers operate outside of academic contexts, because research is always prejudicial and notions of independence and objectivity fictitious. Researchers are always accountable somewhere along the line.

The points made so far indicate that researching disability faces us with a number of problems. How can we ensure that investigations are sufficiently grounded within a social model of disability? What strategies will guarantee that research aims and objectives are not offensive to disabled people? How can we be certain that findings are enabling and not oppressive even in the face of multiple interpretations? How can we be satisfied that research conclusions and outputs will promote disabled people's own interests and priorities? While answers to these questions may not seem particularly elusive, we have found that they are inestimably complicated to deal with in practice. Recognizing that disabled people have to be at the centre of disability research unleashes many troubling questions. Without direct involvement of disabled people, disability research remains ignorant of many issues which are fundamental to the study and is necessarily an arrogant enterprise. But desires to minimize impact of the researcher on the research situation, and to restrict the extent to which those being researched influence the researcher, for example, typify the epistemological challenge.

In the midst of these deliberations are further critical matters concerning rights within the research process. As researchers' understanding of rights and entitlements is very much influenced by their own personal and political experience, we feel that it is necessary to recognize and declare that we are partisan and why. There are various rights that we feel disabled people are entitled to in relation to disability research. A preliminary list includes rights of access to the process of research (planning, carrying out, dissemination), entitlement to set agendas, to describe one's own experiences and to have personal experience valued. Rights to confidentiality, ownership of data, to ask for account to be taken of one's views in implementation of policy and practical changes arising from the research, the right to understand the nature of the research and to challenge and reject research are all important to us, and so will constitute recurring themes throughout the book. We also make reference to the rights of others, such as parents of disabled people; at times it is important to remember that researchers have rights too.

As researchers we have continually addressed the ways in which our work connects with, creates and influences disability. We frequently revisit the role of disabled people in our own disability research. Are the supposedly sacrosanct criteria of, for example, objectivity, validity, generalization and accountability in research compromised if disabled people play a central role in a project? Is there a role for non-disabled researchers in disability studies? Or does the involvement of non-disabled people invariably detract from disabled people's own agendas and create disempowerment? The origins of this complaint are plain enough: if non-disabled researchers are responsible for the legacy of research which has furthered the oppression of disabled people over the years, should they not acknowledge this and vacate the field? Or is it possible to argue that neither disabled people nor their non-disabled peers have to be bound by what has already been done? Can we come to a new understanding in which there is scope for disabled and non-disabled people to carry out research into disability issues together?

Incessant re-examination and reinterpretation of what disability research is intended to achieve will enable researchers to go beyond the legacy of inquiry which has pathologized and oppressed disabled people. We hope that the deliberate reappraisal of our previous research efforts, which is the focus of this book, will encourage readers to reflect upon why we feel that disability research must always be *critical* disability research.

Why we wrote this book

The aims of the book are as follows:

- to place emphasis on progressing a critical approach to disability research
- to illustrate the complexities of dismantling oppression in disability research, illuminated through a critique of traditional positivistic models of inquiry as well as more innovative and reflective ways of doing things
- to provoke commitment to maximizing the relevance of research for equality, inclusion and self-determination of disabled people.

We want to reiterate that we are not trying to provide a specific research philosophy or methodological spirit in which future disability researchers should proceed through this book. Rather we hope to record shifting patterns in our own thinking and to prompt other researchers to reflect critically on attendant implications for their own work.

How this book is organized

The book can be read consecutively or selectively. Each chapter has a short introduction to the context and some of the issues pursued. We give details of a specific research arena and consider how – within that context as individual researchers – we have personally colluded with, or resisted, the recycling of disablement in our investigations. Readers are invited to draw their own conclusions about our collaboration in oppression vs. enablement, and to make links to their own circumstances and obligations. We hope that other researchers may consider, or endorse, the value of working through continual and critical reflection as their projects slowly unfold.

To begin the discussion, in Chapter 2 we expose a variety of oppressive practices which structured a longitudinal observation study of inclusion of d/Deaf[1] children in mainstream primary and nursery settings. This study was designed in the tradition of reductionist research, in which attempts to peel

---

1 As far as possible, the word 'deaf' has been spelt with a lower-case 'd' when it describes the physical condition of deafness, and with a capital 'D' when it refers to the culture of Deaf people. We use the convention 'd/Deaf' as a way of making clear that both those who do, and those who do not, aspire to British Sign Language (BSL) usage and associated cultural heritage are included in the reference.

away bias in interpretation have long been applauded (Bench 1992: 84 and 184). The process of mounting a meticulously objective, reliable and valid research enterprise is described but the need to appraise the usefulness of such parameters becomes patently clear. The focus is on increasing realization that commitment to finding out in traditionally accepted ways can be not only misplaced in disability research, but also dangerous.

In Chapter 3, we review a study of post-school reflections of disabled school leavers commissioned by service providers for the purpose of informing in-schools practice. Emphasis is on developing a collaborative model of inquiry when the researchers and informants both have very little control in relation to those in positions of power. The problem of who has access to the research process is discussed at length. Knowing who your allies are turns out to be an important dimension of research carried out in complex circumstances. The gains that can be made through consultancy with, and representation of, disabled people are made explicit.

Chapter 4 addresses institutional barriers to individual resistance of pressures to reproduce disability through research. As 'insider-researchers', being employees within a family support service under scrutiny, we encountered considerable opposition to positioning service users prominently when it came to deciding what they wanted research to be about. We argue that the priority that *informants* attach to issues explored through any piece of disability research can be used as indices for gauging relevance and utility of the research findings, but describe how the discovery of valuable information and facts can be construed in radically different ways. We examine our personal experience of failed resistance – which led disabled people's interests to be swept aside – in order to encourage readers to build new alliances and, collectively, to affirm and promote the need for critical disability research.

Chapter 5 is structured differently from others and is therefore illustrative of an alternative mode of critical reflection. Instead of analysing one focal project we think more laterally as we consider different research projects which focus in disparate ways on children and disability. Research involving children raises a multitude of ethical, procedural and theoretical controversies connected to the pathologization of childhoods, and these are the focus of this chapter. We address the uncertain position of children's rights in general in society and the effects this has for researchers concerned with disability issues. We believe that children should have the same rights as adults within the research process, but how these can be conveyed in a relevant and appropriate manner, taking into account the age and level of a child's understanding, raises many perplexing questions.

Writing this book has been an uncomfortable process, given the mistakes we have chosen to expose, and in Chapter 6 we hope to clarify how and why we would now wish our disability research to proceed only in certain ways. There were occasions when our feelings about a situation were close to swamping us and only tenacious analysis either at the time or in hindsight enabled us to regather our thoughts and reframe the project rather than giving up altogether. Ultimately we hope that by chasing out some of the skeletons in our own research portfolios, others will consider the merits of continuous reflection on past and present projects. The common and most critical links between all of the chapters concern the power of disability research, and reasons why the observance of disabled people's pivotal role in research which concerns their lives is paramount.

There are problems with the accounts we are presenting, not least because we cannot be certain to protect anonymity and others implicated have no opportunity to reply. We have changed, or avoided, names of agencies and people, but we realize that this is unlikely to safeguard adequately against recognition in every eventuality. We fully accept, and indeed wish to point out, that we present only one version of events in this book. Others who were involved may explain things totally differently, but therein lies the focal challenge of how researchers make sense. By judicious re-examination and juxtaposition of our research experiences we have made invigorating discoveries about the intricacies of critical disability research. We hope that readers might be encouraged to journey likewise.

2

Conventional commitment: traditional research and the creation of disablement

Introduction

For several years now one of the authors has been extremely embarrassed about the piece of disability research which was carried out for satisfactory completion of a PhD (Moore 1993). The work is not embarrassing because it lacks in any scientific or other academic criteria. Indeed the claims it has to conventional objectivity, validity, reliability and the usual dimensions of traditional positivistic social science research are well substantiated. The thesis is packed with adequately defined statistical data, all conscientiously assessed for 'significance' in order to establish statistical conclusion validity. Some researchers would be impressed by the investigator's tenacity in peeling away bias, by the painstaking systematic analysis of quantitative data, and by attempts to see ways in which the findings might be generalized to other populations and situations. The thesis, however, remains a source of considerable unease and as a team we have often reflected upon the extent to which those conducting disability research for a PhD or other qualification can resist demands for their projects to be shaped in ways which are not only 'a waste of time' (Oliver 1992), but also oppressive, both of themselves, and of disabled people being studied.

Close inspection of the project under examination in this chapter reveals how the pursuit of traditional criteria for scientific research may lead to the compilation of a respectable academic PhD thesis, but can also mean that the work undertaken makes absolutely no positive, but plenty of negative, difference to those whose interests it claims to have at heart. Conventional criteria for 'scientific' research can render a disability research project quite meaningless. Potential for oppression of those whose interests the research claims to serve is often actually built into the research by adherence to the usual criteria for scientific credibility. In this chapter it becomes possible to appreciate how the general rules which researchers are still typically required to follow, take away the rights of others through perpetuating myths about the sanctity of a particular type of so-called 'scientific' credibility. It is also important to consider ways in which those in positions of power over a project may have a vested interest in resisting inclusion in the research process of those being researched. In such instances, conventional academic research design comprises an invaluable tool for reinforcing oppression, a theme we revisit throughout the book as alternative approaches are considered.

In this chapter we want to explain by example how established academic thinking about research can steer disability researchers into conducting a project which they might later come to realize has incriminating ramifications. The aim is to encourage disability researchers to develop their awareness of some of the pitfalls associated with traditional ways of doing things. We also wish to show how easily traditional 'scientific' research can be hijacked by those with a vested interest in resisting both inclusive research procedures and implementation of change. Taking a rather uncomfortable look back at a piece of our own research, which we now have to criticize in many respects, may prompt some useful deliberation of why and how disability research needs to be carried out differently.

We begin by outlining the context in which the research took place. Processes of taking stock of the research climate and generally 'getting in' are described next. It becomes important to discuss the emergence of misgivings as a project gradually takes shape. Decisions about making the research appropriate illuminate a need to avoid collusion with pressures for exclusion of disabled children which were always behind this project. Readers can follow the slow realization that those in control of the project may never have intended that the research should be neutral or value free, and then the dawning of an uncomfortable suspicion that the research may have been funded for the purpose of covertly contributing to the marginalization and oppression of disabled people. We look at the difficulties of continuing with a project once researchers realize that they are embroiled in oppressive manipulations, and reflect on subsequent issues involved in disseminating and acknowledging what has been done. It is difficult, and probably invidious, to try to generalize about the role that disabled people should play in disability research but we try to reconcile the issues raised in this chapter with new directions for disabled and non-disabled colleagues working together.

It should be made clear that this review is not intended to judge the competence of individuals involved in the research examined, but to make explicit the complexity of a variety of positions and issues which permeated the research situation.

Thus this chapter aims to

- exemplify and debate the limitations of conventional approaches to researching disability issues
- lay open the pressures researchers often face to work in disabling ways

- acknowledge and explore the personal costs and benefits of reconceptualizing the research enterprise (or of failing so to do) when working in the field of disability studies.

How the study came about

Occasion for the study arose in the context of emphasis placed on inclusion of disabled children in mainstream schools which was established by the 1981 Education Act. As has been well documented elsewhere (Barton 1988; Hegarty 1993; Leadbetter and Leadbetter 1993), the 1981 Act was intended to give legislative effect to the recommendation that opportunity should be made available in the early years for children with impairments to start their education with other children of their own age in mainstream settings. A chance for relevant research arose when, in the context of these initiatives, amalgamation was proposed of a special school for d/Deaf children with two mainstream primary schools. A merger was instituted as the solution when, due to demographic factors, three schools in close geographical proximity met with falling pupil enrolments which threatened their future viability. A junior and an infant school were therefore joined together, and a special school for d/Deaf children closed and replaced by a unit for d/Deaf children attached to the newly combined primary school. Amalgamation was seen to offer increased opportunities for inclusive education, with the same aims for all children. Existing nursery provision for d/Deaf children was extended to create an inclusive preschool facility comprising two classes, for both d/Deaf and hearing children. There was a great deal of optimism about these innovations, and the opening of the new nursery was seized upon as a timely occasion for an evaluative investigation of inclusion to commence.

Looking back, optimism about the prospects for both amalgamation, and subsequently, the potential for productive research was naive. Considerable problems, which might have been predicted, emerged in relation to professional identity and careers for the three heads of schools and their staff, and these were to have a phenomenal impact on both the newly evolving school community and the research process. The day to day running of the project became entangled with school politics, and the general upheaval led some of those in positions of power over the project to seek to manipulate the data in ways which would enhance their own careers and agendas. However, when the researcher embarked on this project she did so as a conventional psychology postgraduate firmly attached to the fantasy of collecting 'objective' data. She presumed that, as researchers take a neutral stance, investigations need not be contaminated by either the personal motives of particular individuals or, in this case, the climate of suspicion and hostility which increasingly came to surround research within the school. Only much later on did it become clear that such faith in objectivity is completely unfounded.

Getting in and taking stock

There were many clues pointing to an ulterior motive behind the willingness of the local education authority's (LEA) to fund this research, but it took a while to put these into a composite picture of what was going on.

Housing of the project within a local teacher training college gave the impression that the LEA was keen to maximize the prospects for objectivity as it seemed to be relinquishing its grip on the everyday running of the project. The project was based alongside the work of an established In-Schools Research Team from the college which was involved in collaborative staff development focusing on management of change in the study school. This, too, seemed to bode well for prospects of implementing change. Involvement in staff development activities meant that a great deal of time would be spent in classrooms over and above that which would be required for the focal research *per se*. In fact, it was through these regular contacts with the staff that the many tensions and conflicting agendas which could affect the research became progressively obvious. It is interesting to look at how, even at this early juncture, the approach to gaining agreement of individual people required to take part in the study, who would ultimately be key stakeholders, was indicative of many of the problems which eventually emerged.

Consent to the project, and to the presence of the researcher in school, was obtained through the school's inspectors and head teachers. Senior personnel expected that teachers and other staff would acquiesce with the project once it had been given the go-ahead at managerial level. Tensions that these sorts of presumptions gave rise to undoubtedly had an impact on emergent data. It is important to recognize that when professionals in positions of power dictate to others that they will be involved in a project, and how, those who do become research participants may not have done so of their own accord.

Fortunately, classroom staff were clear that they themselves valued the prospect of an independent study which could focus on developmental outcomes for the children who were the subject of changing provision. Parents, however, were in an even less powerful position regarding involvement in the study than teachers and classroom assistants. The project was explicitly sanctioned by the professionals who determined entitlement to service provision. It would have taken a brave parent to challenge the right of those same professionals to expect cooperation in an in-service evaluation of their child's experiences, and this militated against freedom for parents to opt out. We return to the role that professionals play in controlling access to parents in Chapter 4, and in governing access to children in Chapter 5. Children, as in most observational studies of this type, were not afforded the privilege of having their consent sought, which meant that some of their fundamental rights within the research process were ignored. Complexities surrounding ways in which children are engaged with disability research are so substantial that we devote the whole of Chapter 5 to this topic.

Those whose consent had been explicitly sought were, then, those who held the greatest power. What was not fully realized was the potency of such a project for the purposes of the most powerful stakeholder, the overseeing LEA inspectorate team. As any reports arising from the project had to be produced under the authority's auspices, the research was to be controlled to suit the LEA's agenda. No doubt this story has great resonance with the experience of other in-service researchers. The purpose of its telling is to prompt those involved in any investigation to reflect on the magnitude of power relations surrounding their work.

Recognizing hidden agendas

In the early stages of setting the project up, background documentation issued to school governors by the LEA suggested that, irrespective of the legislative climate for inclusion described earlier, the principal motivation for amalgamation consisted in falling school rolls over a number of years. More recently Riseborough (1993) has exposed how, in the name of inclusive education, d/Deaf children are often used as part of a 'numbers game' for improving staff:pupil ratios in primary schools. In such situations, it is claimed that d/Deaf children are *'fetishized into things*, a valued additional number from preservational expediency' (Riseborough 1993: 140, emphasis in original). Looking back, this was exactly the position of children who were the focus of the research. It was stressed both in discussions and various school papers that the merger was not brought about by any commitment to inclusion but had coincidentally been forced upon the LEA due to falling admissions. Amalgamation was openly described by the LEA as 'a relatively ad hoc solution' to finding alternatives to segregated provision. In fact, it was publicized that successful development of an inclusive model of provision for profoundly d/Deaf children could not be guaranteed in this instance (Fish Report 1985).

Colleagues from the In-Schools Research Team providing staff development within the school noticed anomalies in the LEA's support of inclusion, pondering in their field notes 'should [the school] bend over backwards to make [inclusion] a success or is it expected to fail? Is the authority's heart in it? Are the conditions right? What are the choices for parents?' They recorded concerns expressed by teachers who wanted to know 'is [inclusion] a cover for doing something on the cheap?' The former special school head had it recorded that in her view d/Deaf children 'could be more usefully and educationally employed through non-integrative activities'. Increased emphasis on inclusion was being structured as an unfortunate by-product of amalgamation, and the venture quickly became characterized by an overall sense of grievance and hostility (Moore 1993). However, for a researcher on the outside looking in, it was possible to view these tensions as a product of the enormity of the undertaking, and to envisage research as potentially helping to identify strengths and commitment, within the study school and their presiding LEA, for pioneering advocacy of universal entitlement for all pupils.

Awareness of a specific hidden agenda came most forcibly, however, when

the LEA provided formal notification that the research must be 'only observation, not about change' (In-Schools Project 1985). The overseeing special
needs inspector insisted that the project be designed to generate data about
developmental outcomes for children which would be 'objective', meaning
uncontaminated by the rumblings of dissatisfaction with prospects for
inclusion increasingly being expressed by staff. It will be plain that pursuit of
this supposed 'objectivity' would actually *guarantee* inadequate insight into
the issues under study, because to assume a position of supposed neutrality
would render the investigator unable to take account of or describe much of
what was going on. Traditionally, however, researchers are advised that
increasing subjectivity, in the sense of reducing the distance between the
observer and the observed (Woolgar 1988), weakens the confidence that
others can have in the findings, and the LEA representative promoted this
view. Those with power over the project intended to exploit widespread
myths about the utility of objectivity in research (Foster and Parker 1995) for
maintenance of the status quo.

Looking back, it is obvious that a more explicit effort to absorb subjective
impressions, rather than to resist them, would have alerted the researcher to
the hidden agendas of those controlling the research. However, through sus-
tained effort to view the research context objectively, which primarily meant
discounting anything anybody said about their experience of changing
schooling, it was possible to persist with the belief that the LEA was committed to the initiative. It seemed far-fetched to construe the LEA's reserve over
accessing the views of classroom staff as an indicator of a desire to boost
prospects for exclusion of hearing impaired children. Reticence could be interpreted as caution since examination of the practical, social or educational
implications of inclusion for d/Deaf children was in its infancy (Webster and
Ellwood 1985; Webster and Wood 1989; D. Edwards 1993). Naturally the LEA
did not confirm the view that its commitment to inclusion was illusory, but it
did fail to deal with issues that seriously undermined the efforts of those
actively pursuing equal access to equal opportunities (Moore 1993).

The potential abuses of the research still seem incredible, but a critical look
back reveals few alternative explanations and others, who were involved at the
time, have been able to confirm this view of what was actually going on. While
the research brief was to evaluate developmental opportunities for children in
inclusive classroom settings, there seemed to be a hidden agenda aimed at promoting segregation, and it appeared as if the research sponsors could ensure
collusion with a divisive view of educational provision for d/Deaf children
through strict adherence to traditional criteria for academic research. Those in
positions of power could allude to the need to retaining objectivity in order to
make sure that the research took no account of the disquiet that staff felt over
levels of support for the venture into inclusive education. No credence was to
be given to how key players felt about the transitions they were part of. The
message imposed upon the researcher was that acceptable research, of which
the LEA might take account, consists in painting a distilled picture of events,
observed in silence, from a vantage point. Explorations from the ground,

attempts to grapple with the essentials of the experiences of central actors and to use provocative interactive exploratory methods which could tap into the rich variety of individual responses to change, all were judged unacceptable by those controlling the investigation, and no further negotiation over methodology could be entered into.

By now many conflicting priorities had been exposed. Educational interests both of d/Deaf children and their hearing peers, needs of teachers and other staff, legitimate concerns of parents, the unrelenting demands of the authority, career prospects for research colleagues in this and other schools, requirements of an Academic Standards Committee ultimately assessing the PhD, plus preservation of some personal sanity, all were priorities which had to be disentangled and safeguarded.

Thinking points

What issues will you be in danger of neglecting if you aim to view your research situation 'objectively'? What will you attempt to discount and why? Whose interests will your investigations best promote if you try to maximize the distance between yourself as a researcher and those who are 'the researched'? How will insight into the research situation be altered if researchers attempt to minimize the distance between those who are the researchers and those who are researched? These questions are important for research generally, but why are they critical for those who research disability matters? How are the issues exacerbated when it comes to disability research?

Conducting an appropriate research enterprise

Despite the level of friction created by the LEA over what the research should consider, those staff involved in the day to day practice of including d/Deaf children and their hearing peers in their classes stayed with their original interest in a profitable exploration of the developmental outcomes for the children who were the subject of changing policy and provision. They were particularly keen to have information about opportunities for communication which inclusive settings might afford d/Deaf children and their hearing peers, and to use this information to stimulate practical ideas about maximizing interactive opportunities for the children for whom they had responsibility. This meant that there did still appear to be the glimmer of possibilities for meaningful research about inclusion which would satisfy the LEA because it did not involve the documentation of anyone's *opinion* about changing provision, but which would also provide some useful material for those children and adults on the receiving end of the changes. Teachers and ancillary staff felt, quite logically, that communication presented the most urgent challenge for everyone involved in inclusion. However, even a relatively innocuous proposal, to design a conventional quantitative longitudinal observation study to detail opportunities for communication, was vulnerable to further manipulations by those seeking to advance a hidden agenda for promoting exclusion.

At the centre of controversy concerning inclusion in the study school was debate over the role of oral/aural (speech) or manual/visual (sign) vehicles in the education of profoundly and severely hearing impaired children. It may seem self-evident that d/Deaf children and their hearing peers will need to share a means of communication, but this issue is complicated by a long history of relentless lack of agreement about what communication methods are feasible and which enable d/Deaf children to establish an easy and effective method of fluent communication (Kittel 1991; Ladd 1991; Bench 1992; Corker 1993; Lynas 1994).

Prior to amalgamation, the school for d/Deaf children held a policy of 'natural oralism', widely interpreted as referring to communication through speaking and listening (e.g. Clark 1989; Lynas 1994). Once amalgamation had taken place, it proved impossible to obtain written confirmation of what the communication policy would now be, but an apparent rhetoric of oralism persisted which, without further clarification of any policy, it was impossible for insiders and outsiders alike to question. This was problematic because specialist staff newly appointed to the unit for d/Deaf children, and many of those from the merging infant and junior schools who would be having contact with d/Deaf children for the first time, felt either intuitively, or based on experience elsewhere, that insistence on speaking and listening would present not only d/Deaf children, but also their hearing peers, with serious communication difficulties. There was no way for teachers, parents, researchers or children to know for certain which means of communication were permissible in the new setting. Not surprisingly perhaps, notes from the In-Schools Research staff development team identified 'a marked gulf' concerning approaches to communication, and a great deal of confusion about appropriate practice.

Thus as new facilities for inclusive provision for d/Deaf and hearing children were opened, the issue of communication, which was both at the heart of the research, and presenting the major challenge to successful implementation of change, was utterly confused. It was not initially realized that ambivalence over communication suited the LEA. This became obvious, however, when eventually it was established that oral/aural (speaking and listening) strategies were to be used with d/Deaf children, but that staff were free to communicate with hearing children in any way which promoted effective communication since hearing children were not subject to restrictive policy and practice.

Ironically then, sign usage was acceptable in communication with hearing children, but not d/Deaf children. When teachers queried this state of affairs, the special needs inspector circulated a letter concluding 'signing seems to me to be a barrier to integration if only because there is no realistic chance that all [staff] can become proficient' (In-Schools Project 1985). Thus difficulties envisaged for staff were reconstituted as children's learning difficulties. The letter implied that 'effective communication seems, to the Authority, to be a barrier to segregation'.

From the beginning it had proved necessary to deal continually with efforts by the LEA to ensure that outcomes would collude with particular ideologies of education and communication for d/Deaf children. The special needs inspector insisted that the project should resist being 'side-tracked' into debates about communication methods otherwise the work would be interpreted as 'getting in the way' (In-Schools Project 1985). It was made clear, through formal channels, that failure to adhere to the LEA's line on communication methods would compromise entitlement to continue the research; this threat had repeatedly to be contested throughout the course of the project. As more restrictions were imposed on what the research might involve, first-hand insights were gained into the potential uses and abuses of research.

Lack of clarity over which methods of communication could legitimately be observed made it necessary to develop a *modality independent* method of analysing children's communication in an effort to avoid conspiracy with the LEA's seemingly transparent attempts to suppress signed interaction and so construct barriers to inclusion. By undertaking to focus on the nature of communicative *intentions* expressed and received by target children, it would be possible to evaluate their opportunities for interaction without explicit reference to how those interactions were conveyed. However, with hindsight, although this aspect of the research design was intended to make any reports as strong as possible, in the sense of maximizing the chances that research outcomes would be seen as credible by the authority, the decision to play down the role of modality in d/Deaf children's experiences of communication shows up considerable shortcomings in methodology which stemmed from lack of consultation with d/Deaf adults. Research that denigrates mode of communication in this field fundamentally denies d/Deaf people their linguistic rights (Montgomery 1986; Jones and Pullen 1992; Corker 1993).

By now, the overseeing school inspector was insistent that consultation with d/Deaf adults on any aspect of the research agenda could not take place. It seemed more evident that the LEA was choosing to militate against the marshalling of any evidence that would defend inclusive models of education. It was as if it wanted a comparatively unequivocal observation study to document reluctant implementation of an inclusion policy by unsupported staff who were being required to disadvantage their most vulnerable pupils. Quite obviously such a project would report back failure and presumably advance the conclusion that d/Deaf children are better off in segregated schools. A PhD thesis, with its attendant publications and presentations at conferences, was presumably expected to confer a certain amount of academic integrity upon the LEA's predetermined argument. Clearly there was explicit danger of colluding with the view that d/Deaf children in mainstream settings are more trouble than they are worth, and the social injustices which research can reproduce were unmistakable.

Readers may visualize how conventional research can promote oppression, particularly if power relations that determine a project are not subject to the most intensive inspection, or if disabled people are left out of the structuring and implementation of studies which regulate aspects of their lives. Disregard of disabled people's own views subverted every aspect of research activity under consideration here, right down to the detail of what the researcher was to observe. This is worth examining in further detail.

Thinking points

What is the role of disabled people in managing power conflicts which surround research? What do you understand by the notion of 'power' in the disability research context, and why is your own particular understanding significant? Who has power over your research activity? What are the interests of those who have such power? How is power being exerted to structure your research activities? Think about how power could be wielded to shape research design as well as procedure, and later dissemination. Can antagonistic power relations be exploited for positive effect? If power relations are oppressive, who are your allies? Who can help you to resist undesirable levels of control over your work?

Structured collusion

We have explained that bimodal communication strategies (speech and sign), while permitted for hearing children, were not to be used with their hearing impaired peers. However, one Deaf child of Deaf parents who were both British Sign Language (BSL) users was to be an exception to this rule. Catherine's parents had insisted on some availability of sign if they were to allow their child to attend the school. Faced with the expensive alternative of funding residential school placement, the LEA relented, and authorized sign usage for this one child, although the LEA failed to back this up with any BSL training or professional support for staff involved. Bimodal communication (the use of speech *and* sign) remained prohibited for all other d/Deaf children. But once sign usage was introduced for Catherine it spread rapidly throughout her classes. Other children, both d/Deaf and hearing, were able to observe bimodal strategies being used with Catherine, and as hearing children were not prevented from using signs, staff could legitimately enable them to interact with her using manual/visual methods.

Hearing children had quickly found that talking to profoundly d/Deaf children produced limited responses, but by using some of the signs they were learning to enable interaction with Catherine, they discovered possibilities for a much more prolific exchange with other d/Deaf children. Hearing and d/Deaf children began to utilize their own, often idiosyncratic, bimodal strategies for enabling them to mutually chat and get along together. Consider the struggle faced by classroom staff who had permission to utilize such resourcefulness in their communicative efforts with only *one* of the d/Deaf children. Their despair was exacerbated by the certain knowledge that although researchers would witness these injustices unfolding, they were not allowed to 'observe' them. This effectively rendered anyone who was concerned without information, and so powerless to take action.

An impossible state of affairs emerged. Sign usage was occurring throughout the nursery. The 40 or so hearing children found it irresistible fun, and effective not only for enabling interaction with their d/Deaf peers, but also for including non-English-speaking hearing children in their conversations and play. Some parents of hearing pupils encouraged their children to attend sign language classes at weekends and began to learn BSL themselves at night school. The parents of another d/Deaf child had noticed that sign usage offered Catherine enriched opportunities for inclusion in classroom life, and demanded that it be made available for their daughter. But the special needs inspector insisted on continuing with the oralist policy for all d/Deaf children except Catherine. The head of the unit for d/Deaf children supported this policy, though the heads of the junior and infant schools within which the unit was amalgamated did not. Thus staff, trying to respond to parents' wishes, and keep up with the naturally emerging bimodal culture for communication in integrated settings, found themselves constantly apprehensive in case they were 'caught' signing by the wrong senior colleague to the wrong child. A few staff stuck to their oralist convictions and the ensuing atmosphere was extremely divisive.

This chaotic situation had a direct impact on the conduct of observational research because the observers had been explicitly directed not to observe any sign usage between staff and d/Deaf children other than Catherine. The rationale seemed to be that if no signing was permitted, then no signed communication could be recorded. Even if the directive was ignored, however, observers were still effectively barred from recording general sign usage because such observations would show staff to be directly going against unit (though not school) policy. The LEA had conceded that sign could be permitted only for Catherine. There was now a dilemma because, if instances of sign usage in interactions with the other d/Deaf children were to be discounted, then the data would necessarily imply that they received fewer and impoverished opportunities for interaction in the inclusive settings as compared with their hearing peers, and would also portray their repertoire of communication strategies as comparatively poor.

At this point earlier suspicions seemed incontrovertible. The purpose of operationalizing a highly structured, theoretically objective observational research study of communication in inclusive settings, which was deliberately manipulated to neglect full account of possible communication strategies available, was to produce a picture of inclusion as offering no developmental advantages for d/Deaf children. The conclusion would be that inclusion was not working. Those funding the project were determining what could and what could not be observed, and in so doing, regulating the experiences of disabled children according to their own predilections. It was then discovered that a nationally known advocate of oralism and of highly specialized segregated education for hearing impaired children was in a strong position of influence over the project, indicating that vested interests in research outcomes were not imaginary.

Dissemination and implementation of change

Classroom staff wanted to know if availability of bimodal strategies was enhancing opportunities for communication for the children in their classes, and they wanted feedback on whether anything they were doing was improving the children's experiences of inclusion. The researcher had either to distort the findings, and report no insight into bimodal interactions, or to report the real situation. Deciding to disclose what was actually going on would dramatically affect prospects for dissemination, because emergent data would compromise the professionalism of many staff who knew they were operating outside of the rules of their institution.

Eventually it was decided that the immediate interests of the children at the centre of the investigation could not be subjugated but had to be treated as paramount. The decision was taken to produce a holistic account of the children's experiences of communication, without discounting crucial evidence. Consequently, it would be possible to provide off the record feedback only to those school staff who had shown themselves to be disabled people's allies by accepting initiatives for sign language and seeking a role for d/Deaf adults and their representative agencies. Production of an end of project report would have to be avoided and writing up of a PhD thesis was (at least initially) suspended. Implementation of change in the study school would be minimal because there could be no risk of exposing staff who had sought to support d/Deaf children with signed communication; this problem constituted a further source of oppression. Since the research conclusions could be only cautiously divulged, those who might benefit most from the findings would probably never actually see them.

This was frustrating for a researcher who had started out with optimistic ambitions to report on radical changes for improving the education and development of d/Deaf children. Two years' twice weekly observation in the study school had suggested tangible and specific directions for enhancing the experience of young d/Deaf children and their hearing peers in inclusive settings, but seemed destined to make no difference. Yet trends indicated by the data were believed to be very important. For instance, it could be shown that availability of a bimodal culture bears enormous positive influence upon both d/Deaf and hearing children's experiences of communication, and subsequently enriches their experiences of inclusion. It was shown that sign usage in the classroom makes a direct impact on initiations that children engage in, on responses they make, on their own modes of communication, on their use of referential acts, on interpersonal aspects of their communication and on social contexts in which children find themselves. The data provided strong evidence that bimodal strategies had a substantial and enriching impact on children's styles of interaction, with direct implications for their personal and social well-being in inclusive environments. It was, however, impossible to set up in-service training initiatives on the basis of these more or less illicit findings. Even though it was possible to avoid dissecting styles of adult interaction directly, it was impossible to safeguard individual members of staff and so the interests of children were jettisoned.

d/Deaf children in the study school were, without doubt, disabled by a particular model, held by non-disabled professionals, of what communication should be. Implementation of an oralist policy grounded the inclusion of d/Deaf children in a set of assumptions about equality and sameness that assigned disability to them. Such a process ensures that deficit views of d/Deaf children's communication abilities are corroborated. The resistance to difference, which underpins oralist philosophy, provides a means of justifying implementation of oppressive communication policies in the education of d/Deaf children. It was difficult to conduct enabling research in the study school because those in power shaped the enterprise in order to recycle their personal convictions concerning oralism and exclusion, and steadfastly refused to consider d/Deaf people's own ideas for priorities and insights (Ladd 1988; Corker 1993).

Despite the innumerable problems which beset the project, it had been possible to collect sensible data which generated practical indications for enhancing the experience of d/Deaf children in integrated settings; however, this information could not be properly disseminated. Frustrations surrounding the limited prospects for acting on the information obtained were shared by all of the school staff who had accommodated the strain of continual observations into every aspect of their work for the sole purpose of enhancing their classroom practice. At the point when it became obvious that, despite having funded an intensive three year investigation, the LEA would not even engage in discussions about emergent implications concerning sign language and the role of d/Deaf adults in schools, one teacher, who had invested most in stimulating understanding of bimodal communication strategies, resigned.

This meant that part-way through the research, a newly trained replacement teacher was appointed. Through no small coincidence, the new appointee had an oralist background and was unsympathetic to the view that sign could provide the key to meaningful participation in classroom life. This placed the new member of staff at odds with her own classroom assistant and in opposition to the teacher in charge of hearing children whom she would work alongside. As everyday inclusive activities became more difficult to manage given the divergence of views and continued lack of support from the LEA, d/Deaf pupils were increasingly taken out of the interactive milieu of inclusive classes for the purposes of specialist oralist training in segregated settings. The LEA had thus won its battle to perpetuate exclusion of d/Deaf children and to oppress the language and culture of d/Deaf people. Even though the researcher had managed to resist the most blatant attempts to manipulate the research process for these ends, it was impossible to withstand the LEA's level of control over research findings.

The personal costs of admitting to such a state of affairs proved very high. It was impossible to write a PhD thesis which could be seen by the LEA, and without its endorsement of an end of project report, a thesis could not be submitted. Three years' work resulted in no report.

Role of disabled people in the research

The obvious strategy for decreasing the likelihood that the research would prove so fruitless would have been to involve d/Deaf consultants in the project. As explained, the possibility of doing so met with immediate disapproval by the special needs inspector in whose view involving d/Deaf adults would compromise the legitimacy of the research (the reader will recognize the pitfalls of unremitting investment in the mythical properties of 'objectivity'). For a hearing researcher, the exclusion of d/Deaf people created a great deal of insecurity because, without their central involvement, it was inevitable that the research exercise would remain ignorant of many issues relevant to d/Deaf children's experiences. Failure to build in a platform for d/Deaf people to influence this project, though not of the researcher's own volition, rendered the study at best, an arrogant enterprise, completely divorced from the agenda of those with personal experience of both hearing impairment and exclusion.

Owning up and personal costs

As the longitudinal observation period finished and the research drew to a close it became obvious that an end of project report could not be presented to the school, causing widespread despondency. The LEA, the school and the research team were all dissatisfied with the evident lack of outcomes from the project, albeit for different reasons. The LEA had no research publications commending its philosophies and practices, the school had no evidence with which to challenge policy or develop practice, and the researcher had no prospect of a PhD. These considerations are relatively unimportant, however, in comparison to intense disablement produced by the whole episode for d/Deaf children and the wider community of disabled people and their allies.

Disappointment with the lack of research outcomes, openly expressed by school staff, could only partially be allayed through taking in cakes and wine in one or two bleak attempts to engineer a friendly exit. Various efforts, such as volunteering to make videos of residential field visits and weekend concerts, were made to somehow 'compensate' parents and teachers for what appeared to them as the researcher's failure to tell them anything useful. Some data were shared with one of the teachers undertaking a Diploma in

Special Educational Needs, but she too was powerless to broadcast emergent findings beyond the submission of revealing essays which she had hoped might be assessed by a lecturer who was also one of the school governors. However, the lecturer concerned, who was known to be a personal friend of the special needs inspector, managed to evade the critical pieces of course work by suggesting that, in the interests of fairness, the teachers' reports should be assessed by someone without school connections.

School staff had been willing to share inside information in the hope that research would help them enhance prospects for successful inclusion. They had been open and honest about the frustrations of coping with the reality of implementing change, the day to day effort of working with colleagues who felt differently from them about what was happening, and about the exhausting task of coping with continually conflicting messages from management about how things should be done. Even though such insights had not been solicited for research purposes, access to a variety of information, beyond the disregarded observation data, further contributed to the reseacher's abject sense of failure.

An important lesson for other disability researchers is to acknowledge that, and try to understand how, once you are in situ you are no longer the sole determinant of your own identity or actions (Woolgar 1993; Connors and Glenn 1996). It is crucial to think about how power can be taken back, if needs be, in order to advance your own plans for the research. For non-disabled researchers this is obviously an area where disabled co-researchers could prove invaluable allies, and in some situations the reverse will also be true. An immensely complicated set of boundaries determines relations between the researcher and the researched; these need to be mediated and adapted to ensure that those being researched in disability studies, have sufficient recourse to advocacy. If, like the child subjects within this study, they are not in a position to be self-advocates, then the case for conferring with other disabled people is unequivocal.

Conclusions

Trying to maintain distance as an observer, as in the case of the research described in this chapter, does *not* ensure that a truer image of events and practices will be assembled, but can yield restrained, and possibly corrupt, research outputs. In any research context where disabled people and their representative agencies are potentially oppressed or made vulnerable, it is clearly preferable for researchers to reflect on ways of avoiding this and, wherever possible, to accentuate the role of disabled people themselves in resistance. If disabled people are to be intentionally denied access to the research process, as in the study under discussion, then it is essential that researchers do not gloss over the fact that ensuing inadequacies in their work may well invalidate their research productions.

Several years after funding for the research had ended, the LEA representative who had in the eyes of d/Deaf parents and their allies, been principally associated with upholding barriers to inclusion, retired. Eventually the project was sufficiently forgotten for it to be written up. With hindsight, and a great deal of support from disabled researchers, it became possible to understand much of what had gone on in terms of the politics of disablement through research, such as we have tried to unravel here, and this provided some scope for returning to and at least beginning to deal with the considerable short-comings of the work.

The principal lessons for other researchers consists in recognition of the pressures that researchers face to work in disabling ways. Through other research examples presented in this book, we try to suggest how researchers can move from recognizing these pressures to resisting them; we continue to find this a difficult and disturbing process. Recognition of the dominant and oppressive relations which encircle research activity is not straightforward or uncomplicated and there is always the dangerous temptation of refuge within a variety of research which could be so. Recognizing the enormity of personal and political, structural and institutional factors which surround one's under-takings more often than not reinforces a sense of powerlessness and instils despondency. Although we and others (Stevenson and Cooper 1997) argue that reflexivity is an essential component of research it does not in itself pro-vide the key to dismantling disabling barriers in research. These cannot merely be thought away; from thoughts must follow action.

Thinking points

What pressures are you facing to conduct research in disabling ways? Can you identify the source(s) of such pressure, and in so doing, begin to think about ways of resisting? What are the personal costs for you if you fail to engage with the resistance of oppression in your research? On the other hand, what are the benefits of deciding so to do? Can you recognize ways in which taking a conventional approach to research might limit your insight into disability issues? What can you do to bring about change? Who might offer you support for this?

3

Divided commitment: researching with service users and providers

Introduction

At the end of Chapter 2 we had begun to reconceptualize the nature of the research enterprise. In the field of disability studies, researchers cannot afford to approach their projects in the traditional mode of objective, value free inquiry. Instead, it is critical to recognize the potential of conventional research activity for reproducing, and even creating, disablement and oppression. Having recognized this, prospective disability researchers should maximize the extent to which their activities promote the rights of disabled people within the research process and also to continue to reflect upon this at every stage.

The project that is the focus of this chapter attempts to illustrate how, through our own research efforts, we tried to progress beyond recognizing the role that research can play in perpetuating disability, and to resist pressures to work in disabling ways. Unfortunately, we only partially succeeded in accomplishing this, most significantly perhaps because, as in many applied research situations, a complex web of conflicting priorities was quickly uncovered. The problem of how those in positions of power over a project can control prospects for assertion, or conversely denial of, the rights of those being researched, is found to be inescapable.

The purpose of this chapter is to alert researchers to critical issues involved in managing the priorities of all those in the research field, in order to maximize access to the research process for disabled people who are the focus of the study. This is not a straightforward business, as we hope the central project story will reveal. We have been led to think about whether disabled people are any different from other subjects of research with regard to rights within the research process. We have concluded that the notion of rights *is* different for disabled people in this context in respect of the minority status they are afforded within society, as evidenced by the 1995 Disability

Discrimination Act. In our view, it is important to develop a heightened profile of the rights of disabled people to express their views, because identification with minority and oppressed groups impinges on a person's right to be heard by the majority. We have attempted to depict the practical implications of these issues in this critique.

This chapter aims to

- illustrate the obstacles that researchers may face in trying to optimize disabled people's rights to self-determination
- discuss the difficulties of resistance when efforts to work in empowering ways are potentially thwarted
- prompt further consideration of how researchers can increase meaningful representation of disabled people in research.

We start by outlining the context in which the research took place.

The focus for this chapter is a study concerning the post-school reflections of disabled school leavers. The work was conducted by two of the authors in collaboration with service providers in order to inform in-schools practice (Moore and Beazley 1995). It was an endeavour to carry out a research inquiry that would benefit young d/Deaf people through investigating any aspect of the role of a service for post-16 students with hearing impairment which key service providers identified as of interest. Our motivations for doing this project deserve some attention first, as it is important for researchers to recognize their own reasons for becoming involved in a particular project and any potential or actual influence these may have on the activity as a whole (P. Shakespeare *et al.* 1993).

Initially, the two of us involved in this project were instructed to work together by our head of department, who was increasingly under pressure to promote recognition of the department through research activity and associated publications (P. Shakespeare *et al.* 1993). We were therefore constrained to produce some material research outputs. At the time, one of us had recently emerged from the difficult research experiences described in Chapter 2, and the other was relatively new to carrying out applied investigations in the field. Thus, we were a combination of one determined to promote enablement through research, and one optimistic about the possibility of so doing. We shared an interest in working with hearing impaired children and so decided to explore possibilities for collaborative research with the local Service for Hearing-Impaired Children.

We approached the research with several priorities. Experience of the disabling potential of inquiry meant that we were increasingly mindful of how problems can be created if research does not promote the interests of those whose work involves day to day contact with disabled people. We were also obliged to protect an already long-standing clinical link with service providers. Thus we opted to liaise directly with teachers, rather than those in greater or lesser positions of power within the service. Working with teachers should offer good possibilities for advancing the interests of d/Deaf pupils and school leavers. We made the assumptions that, as teachers were in daily contact with young disabled people, they might be committed advocates for current and former pupils, and that the voices of teachers might carry more weight with senior management than the voices of pupils and school leavers themselves. Later we came to realize that we had grossly oversimplified issues involved in promoting the rights of disabled people within research, particularly the rights to self-determination and self-advocacy.

As the study commenced we knew that teachers were embroiled in familiar controversies concerning educational provision for d/Deaf pupils (Webster and Wood 1989; D. Edwards 1993), and we prepared to take this into account. We knew, for example, that the local authority was in a state of flux with moves afoot to introduce some form of signing into what, until then, had been a staunchly 'oral' service adhering to a policy of no use of sign. In addition, the segregated 'special' school system was in the process of closing down and a policy for greater inclusion only relatively newly in place. As we had considerable experience of both communication and inclusion issues we hoped to be able to implement beneficial change through research (Barton and Clough 1995) in this context. However, we knew little of local service management structures and style, nor of the relations between the local Deaf community and the service, whereas these factors ultimately turned out to be the key determinants of prospects for change.

Getting started

At the start of this project we were anxious to facilitate regular input from d/Deaf people. Hearing impaired people were increasingly expressing anger about the violation of their experiences by hearing researchers (Pullen and Jones 1992) and we knew from the outset that we had to be vigilant about whose priorities our research activities would actually be promoting. We knew that as non-disabled researchers working alongside non-disabled service providers we would be extremely limited in the extent to which we could hope to make sense of issues that affect the lives of disabled people. However, we were not in a position to offer funding for a co-researcher, and were worried about obvious exploitation involved in inviting any d/Deaf person to join the project without remuneration.

We compromised on a strategy whereby we invited three members of the local Deaf community to participate in a series of regular advisory meetings. We tried to reduce our anxieties about not funding attendance at these meetings through setting up fee-paying sign language courses for students within our university, in order to generate some paid employment for the advisers, albeit generating only an unrelated source of income. We also made periodic contact with a Deaf researcher who had worked on another project with young d/Deaf people and were able to incorporate her views on the project with particular reference to specific details of design and methodology. Our worries about not adequately involving d/Deaf people in the research were partially allayed by the view of the advisers, who felt that the absence of a d/Deaf co-researcher would not necessarily devalue any information we, as hearing researchers, were able to obtain from d/Deaf people taking part in this study. We gladly accepted this concession at the time, as we needed to get started; however, we knew that our Deaf advisers were offering us friendship and personal support in order to allay our misgivings. They realized that attempting to further break down barriers to their participation in the project would endanger prospects for research of any kind going ahead. Opportunities for inclusion, and representation of disabled people's own concerns in the project, were seriously curtailed because the collaborating service providers insisted upon keeping the involvement of d/Deaf people tokenistic.

Against this background we began to have regular meetings with teachers from the local service that we were working with in order to establish research objectives and to decide upon proposed methodology. The service providers felt it unnecessary to involve the Deaf advisers in these discussions. This meant that the project was shaped by ideas which came originally from hearing service providers and which were commented upon later, and separately, by Deaf people. This was the first point at which we began to realize that despite our intentions to promote the interests of d/Deaf people through this research, any interests they held would be marginalized, and it was those of non-disabled people that were actually coming first. Nevertheless, we persisted with working in this way because retaining some contact with the Deaf advisers was critical to us personally; at the very least, we felt that setting up the consultancy group had provided some scope for forging direct links between Deaf adults and the service. The main feature that we strongly wished to underpin the research, was that it should be *collaborative* at as many levels as possible and so we wanted both to appease the service providers, and to smooth a path towards active involvement with the service for the Deaf advisers.

We hoped that maximizing collaboration would help to ensure that the research was beneficial to d/Deaf service users as well as providers, and not simply conducted to enhance the credibility of professionals, including, in this respect, ourselves. Through collaboration with service providers we hoped to avoid the pitfalls of much previous educationally based research which has presented service providers with negative findings about aspects of their work that they may not themselves define as central. That all concerned were mindful of the potentially damaging impact of research can clearly be seen from the emphasis we placed in a letter to the teachers involved:

> we share your concern that the service would not wish us simply to 'do some research and then go away' and would like to reiterate that we will only wish to move forward after close consultation and in ways which the service identifies as useful.

The trouble with these remarks is that they expressly exclude reference to d/Deaf people's own perspectives on the research agenda. In the name of maximizing cooperation, we were being seduced into not causing controversy and so found ourselves trying to be philosophical about the lack of any early indication that service users were to be involved in crucial decisions about the research process. We accepted that if the project was to lead to better educational practice, only those who could take full account of the realities of the context could truly recognize the issues to explore, but had hoped service providers would wish to include recommendations from young d/Deaf people about what goals might be set. However, while we were happy enough that the research questions would be generated from inside the service, it was not the case that service providers themselves prioritized the interests of service users. Increasingly we came to realize that positive change for d/Deaf people was construed as a secondary outcome of the research in the minds of service providers, for whom the primary objective was to advance their own ideas about service development. This state of affairs soon stifled the task of evolving appropriate research methodology as will be seen in the next section.

Thinking points

How can you involve disabled people in your research activity? A variety of roles can be allocated to secure involvement of disabled people in research. The terms 'co-researchers', 'collaborators', 'advisers' and 'consultants' are used interchangeably . . . but how do these definitions alter prospects for a person's rights within the research process? Whose voice is heard is of fundamental concern here. What difference does the way in which disabled people contribute to a research project make?

Research design

After a while, three areas of interest for an interview-based inquiry were decided upon:

- factors which contribute to 'success' for young d/Deaf people at the post-16 stage
- the communicative effectiveness and interpersonal skills of recent school leavers
- possibilities for involving d/Deaf adults in the work of the post-16 service.

On reflection it is interesting to note that although interlinked, the first issue was actually that prioritized by service providers, the second reflected the interest in personal empowerment of young d/Deaf people held by the researchers, and the third issue stemmed from the interests of the Deaf advisers. The issues were interwoven in the spirit of working together collaboratively but, in the light of a careful look back, can be seen separately to promote quite different objectives. Had we explicitly acknowledged the separateness of the focal issues at the time, some of the eventual difficulties that arose for reconciling the various participating parties to the research outcomes might have been reduced. While we appeared to have negotiated a shared research agenda, in reality we had only loosely stitched together a bag of mixed priorities, and so were necessarily destined to serve the interests of each participating party inadequately. None of the research issues was decided by those whose interests the research was supposed to be about, namely young d/Deaf school leavers themselves.

Nevertheless, the three issues listed above were agreed to be of mutual interest, and the next task was to set about researching them in ways which we hoped would recognize the rights of young d/Deaf people who used the service. However, prospects for promoting the interests of service providers, over and above those of service users, came more to the fore as teachers overseeing the project exerted control first over selection of prospective interviewees and second over what interviewees might be given the opportunity to discuss.

Whose views are worth having?

Access to young d/Deaf people connected with the post-16 service had to be gained through service providers. We made tentative suggestions about selection processes, offering for example to include all school leavers within a particular cohort, or proposing methods of random sampling, but the post-16 teachers felt that they knew best which young people it would be appropriate to invite to take part. Initially they expressed reservations about communication processes, construing the 'problem' of easy and effective communication between interviewer and interviewee as one that legitimately excludes some people from participation in the research process. We resisted this rather transparent attempt at exclusion until, eventually, it was agreed that all prospective interviewees could be offered the opportunity of having a sign language interpreter present during the interview. None of the young people whom the post-16 teachers had decided to approach had been given the opportunity to use interpreters in school; it was not surprising when none requested this particular resource.

We felt rather despondent because if the primary form of communication used in the interviews was, after all, to be speech with the written form and some gesture used as a back-up, there was some justification if service providers nominated only interviewees whom they felt would cope with an interview based predominantly on the communication methods of the hearing world. Clearly this would structure the research project in ways which members of the Deaf community would find oppressive. In relation to the central research issues, 'factors leading to "success" for young d/Deaf people at the post-16 stage' would be accessed only for those deemed by service providers to be *oral* successes; insights into 'the communicative effectiveness and interpersonal skills of recent school leavers' would similarly be ascertainable only from those deemed to be *oral* successes; and thus 'possibilities for involving d/Deaf adults in the work of the post-16 service' could be presented as negligible.

We were extremely anxious *not* to exclude participants on the grounds of their communication strategies and so proposed an interview procedure whereby we would work as a pair, with one of us assigned responsibility for 'enabling communication'. We are aware that there are many complex issues surrounding mediated interactions which we (Beazley *et al.* 1997a; 1997b) and others (Moorehead 1997) have discussed elsewhere. In consequence, although we were conscious that some degree of compromise might be involved, we wanted to avoid mediation and to maximize direct communication. As part of this we made further effort to avoid over-reliance on spoken language during the course of interviews and planned parts to be focused around pictures we asked respondents to draw. This technique had been used by one of the researchers in a previous project where it was found that drawing pictures greatly enriched the respondents thinking around focal topics and their ability to express themselves, as well as breaking down power barriers created by the interview situation (Rose *et al.* 1986). These suggestions were accepted by service providers since the qualifications and communication skills of one of the researchers as a specialist speech and language therapist could not be denied; we were therefore able to ensure that perceived level of oral communication skill did not become the main criterion for selection of young d/Deaf people to take part in the research. We felt that this struggle had yielded a glimmer of recognition for the right to be heard for the young d/Deaf school leavers connected with the service.

The next task was to write an introductory letter which service providers would forward to potential participants. Two of the Deaf advisers checked the letter for appropriate language content, which gave some scope for ensuring that research objectives were regarded as sensible by d/Deaf people. Beyond this point we had to relinquish control over selection and description of the project aims to those in the gatekeeping role. We were not able to ensure open access to participation either through who was approached in the first place, or through how the project and ourselves were portrayed. This particular aspect of delegation was (and always is of course) risky in terms of the researchers' ability to ensure equal access to participation. However, the project was going forward and the interviews were now in the process of being arranged.

Thinking points

In what ways can researchers ensure the rights for disabled people as potential participants (a) to have the project ideas presented in an accessible form (b) to agree or decline to take part (c) to deal with the chosen methodology? How might researchers need to modify procedures, where their own communication skills may otherwise be inadequate to support full access for some disabled people to the research process?

Who decides what is worth knowing?

Having negotiated a shaky course for recruiting participants and engaging them in the research process, another area of controversy emerged concerning *what* participants could contribute to the project. We envisaged that interviews should be designed to enable interviewees to retain maximum control over what they chose to contribute, although it is well known that research relationships can never be entirely balanced (T. Shakespeare 1996). The Deaf advisers and ourselves wanted the interview to provide young d/Deaf people with an opportunity to put forward their own post-school concerns and reflections, and for their disclosures to be shaped by their own interests rather than by those of service providers. Thus, our emphasis was on the right to self-determination. In addition, we wanted the process of taking part in a research interview to provide the young d/Deaf participants with some tangible personal benefits, and so hoped to build in possibilities for respondents to increase self-awareness and to reconceptualize aspects of their current situation and plans for the future if they wished to do so. This approach had been found extremely useful by one of the researchers in a study of personal and social education with hearing school leavers (Rose *et al.* 1986).

We were set on the interview being based on the social model of disability with the focus being on identifying disabling barriers and ways of dismantling them. This led us to plan semi-structured interviews which could provide participants with the opportunity to recall their experiences of preparation for leaving school, and re-examine elements of their experience which they defined as important. Interviewees could be invited to reflect on their current situation, and also to focus on their future and consider strategies for achieving long term goals and objectives. Prompts were built in to enable the young people to think about what and whom would help or have helped them to surmount obstacles and achieve goals. Given the high degree of personal exploration envisaged, we were concerned about the pitfalls of the one-off interview which can leave the respondents with many unanswered questions. To deal with this, we followed the suggestion of the Deaf Research Consultant, and invited participants to take part in a follow-up group discussion.

Misunderstanding arose from the fact that these plans departed from conventional question–answer routines because service providers interpreted our lack of specific directives as an indication that we did not know what we wanted the interviewees to discuss. Our concern not to impose a research agenda left us appearing vague and seemingly without clear ideas of our own, and understandably met with some apprehension. The post-16 teachers could see the relevance of open-ended in-depth explorations, but were concerned that such interactions would not end up by telling the service what the service wanted to know. There was some difficulty in managing our divergent perspectives here, because our priority had always been to reflect back what young d/Deaf people wanted service providers to know, and this is quite different, of course, from finding out what service providers wanted to discover. We anticipated a struggle at this point, over the eventual nature of the interview procedure, and dreaded being directed to ask interviewees specific questions in particular ways as we felt that such an approach would be inherently disempowering.

The temptation to put forward our own ideas had been great as the necessary reserve we had to show as researchers conflicted sharply with our need to satisfy our social role within the context. The latter role inclined us to offer suggestions in order to be cooperative, supportive and facilitative as well as to look informed. The potentially tense nature of the process was helped by a number of things. First, both sides seemed to have a shared desire to partake in a project. Second, we had prior positive experience of each other in quite different roles, and as others have pointed out (P. Shakespeare *et al.* 1993), often people will assume that if *you* are all right then the research will be all right. Third, we all endeavoured to make the social setting for the research meetings as positive as possible.

The role of the obligatory cup of tea and affable enquiries about families and weekends should not be underestimated for establishing some ongoing commitment in a new research enterprise. While this may seem a superficial practicality to raise, it is important for researchers to be aware of the dilemmas posed by trying to match research and social roles and also to separate out the two parts, identifying the contradictory and complementary aspects of each. Sometimes the business of a planned meeting was swamped by polite overtures, but substantial efforts to ease tensions and embarrassments did considerably reduce the risk of the project being jettisoned. We continually tried to reaffirm our commitment to working collaboratively towards beneficial outcomes for the service. Suddenly, much to our surprise, we were given the go-ahead to proceed in whichever way we liked. In confident moments we felt that our strategy of always consulting with our Deaf advisory group had paid off, lending some credibility to our preferred methodological approach. In weaker moments we feared the post-16 teachers had simply decided that we were incapable of conducting a meaningful research enterprise and had opted to get the project over with as quickly as possible. By now our relationship with the service felt precarious and, as the project went on, undercurrents that we already in part had detected, became more ominous.

The reality of initial doubts about our competence was revealed nearly twelve months later by one of the teachers orchestrating the project, who wrote 'it is true that my misgivings about the methodology for the research were proved misplaced to the extent that an interesting and potentially useful report did ensue'.

'An interesting and potentially useful report'

This comment shows that service providers were not overly impressed by the utility of the research, despite all our efforts to address practical and policy relevance on their terms. The origins and significance of this problem merit further examination.

The first indication that service providers were not pleased to be uncovering the young d/Deaf people's views began to emerge even as the data were being collected. While there was agreement that confidentiality of the interviewees would always be strictly respected, service providers sometimes tried to use their knowledge of those involved to guess who might have said what or, on occasions, actually asked some of those whom they had nominated what had been discussed. We surmised that where service providers felt uncomfortable about issues arising, they sought to challenge the validity of the contributions being given. While interviews were still in progress we found service providers were trying to distance themselves from emergent criticism by reminding us that the interviewees had come from a range of different school services and by mentioning that some of them were unlikely to be mature enough to know their own minds. We realized that if what the young d/Deaf people wanted to say did not comply with the expectations of service providers then their views were to be undermined and disparaged. Our impression was confirmed when one of the post-16 teachers wrote to say 'we [are] unhappy that you appeared to take everything the students say at face value' and asked us 'to include in the [report] a note disclaiming such an attitude'. This is in contrast to the more enlightened disposition noted by Marks (1996) whereby in a number of studies 'senior teachers and administrators have been impressed by [pupils'] perception and good sense' (Marks 1996: 115).

Despite the inference that the reflections of some of the young d/Deaf participants should be discounted, our own confidence in what they were revealing was high. We had built in to the interviews a check of how participants felt about their own contribution, not least because the interviews clearly departed from the usual question–answer routine and may have raised issues for the respondents that they had not considered before. We were satisfied that interviewees regarded the discussions as a positive, thought-provoking experience, and that they valued, and responded well to, the opportunity to think hard about the contexts in which they were, and might be, in the future. All this meant that the business of presenting the research findings was bound to be complicated because service providers sought to invalidate many of the reflections of the young d/Deaf people, whereas we accepted their validity. Service providers were always in the position of being able to imply 'yes, but we have known [the young d/Deaf participants] for *x* number of years, whereas you did only meet them once or twice'. So, by the time the personal interviews and the group discussion were completed and we set about producing a draft report, there were various indications which augured how it would be received (Moore and Beazley 1995).

Responses to the report were mixed. Service providers were the first to see it and were given the chance to request amendments. Still, their response was guarded. While we had anticipated this reserve, it added considerable tension to what was already a strained situation. However, we took account of their criticisms, adding four appendices with notes which the post-16 teachers maintained clarified issues about the support service's provision. The requested amendments were obviously intended to distance the service from comments made by young d/Deaf people with which they did not agree. That we acquiesced to this inclusion reflects the degree of accountability we felt to the service providers as researchers with professional ties to retain. Once again, we realized that the young d/Deaf participants had been marginalized, particularly as we had not sought suggested amendments from them at the draft report stage. In our endeavours to remain answerable to the service that commissioned the work, we had surrendered accountability to service users.

On a more positive note, the Deaf advisers were delighted with the report and requested that copies be sent to a number of national societies for d/Deaf people with the aim of reaching a wider audience through their magazines. One of the advisers, who worked for a national charity, set about trying to get his group to publish the whole report. The enthusiasm shown by the Deaf advisers for making the views of the young d/Deaf people more widely known, together with the importance that the young d/Deaf people had themselves attached at the group meeting to trying to provide more people with insights into their situations, refuelled our commitment to them by making sure the research did have an impact, and did not just evaporate following circulation of the report. We reminded ourselves of our original aim which had been to carry out research which would make a positive difference to all of the major stakeholders – teachers and post-16 service providers, young d/Deaf people, and representatives of the adult d/Deaf community. We still harboured a fantasy that the research activity might act as a catalyst for forging links between the three groups, and so decided to instigate further discussion of project findings with the service.

Making an impact

Our continued endeavours to keep on good terms with service providers, and their desire that some profit could be obtained from having authorized the interviews, helped to establish a forum for further discussion of how the project might benefit the service. It had been difficult for the post-16 teachers to accept the report wholeheartedly but there was some recognition that there were messages which needed to be passed on to others. We were greatly encouraged when they invited us to join the full team of staff for a training day to share the findings, give an opportunity for discussion and provide a chance for practice and policy changes to emerge. This invitation seemed to indicate support from the post-16 teachers and their managers for both project and report, and since initial responses to our work had been rather hostile, we were relieved to receive this sign of recognition.

A view which had been frequently expressed by the d/Deaf interviewees was that young people such as themselves could usefully work alongside teachers supporting pupils in school. They felt that they could assist teachers to consider new avenues for smoothing the transition from school to work or further/higher education. Since this idea came from the critical stakeholder group, and it matched the interest of the Deaf advisory group in exploring possibilities for involving d/Deaf adults in the work of the post-16 service, we hoped that it might comprise the focus for the training session. This conjecture promptly brought us into more tension with the post-16 teachers.

The post-16 staff had a clear idea of what they wanted from the session: a half-hour lecture on contents of the report and then discussion restricted to three issues which *they* had identified as the main ones. We did not want to waste the limited time available in going through the details of the project when this information was already available in the report. After some debate about the possibility of allowing teachers themselves to identify the challenges that the findings raised for them, and then using the session to focus on finding ways of implementing change, we were somewhat reluctantly given permission to plan the session along these lines instead. We forwarded a programme and an appropriate number of copies of the report to be circulated for reading by those who would be attending, prior to the training day.

We had considered asking some of the young d/Deaf people themselves to be involved but decided, given the reluctance of the post-16 teachers to accept their contributions, that this might put them in an uncomfortable position. This endeavour to protect the research participants, without giving them the right to choose, was misplaced because it left us as non-disabled researchers trying to represent the views of disabled people. We were finding it difficult to resist ways in which service providers could wield their power to regulate the degree of input which young disabled people could make to the project, and allowing our original emphasis on promoting self-determination of disabled people to be diluted.

Although we had decided not to involve young d/Deaf people in presenting the session, we aimed to facilitate thinking among teachers about practical ways of responding to the young people's reported reflections at both an individual level and a wider group level. We planned to focus on individual action plans and the development of a group agenda for implementing change, assuming that, as experienced tutors, we could keep the concerns of d/Deaf school leavers in central view. But here we own up to yet another questionable decision in retrospect. Retaining control over dissemination for ourselves would inevitably contribute to disempowerment of the researched.

We should have foreseen that without the presence of d/Deaf school leavers at the training session, it would be easy for the focus to slide away from their needs, and back to the all too familiar problems that teachers encounter. Strong feelings emerged about major stresses at work resulting from being under-resourced. A sense of powerlessness was uncovered because teachers felt that they had insufficient time to provide adequate liaison, to consider ways of extending or changing their service provision or to implement any new ideas. Emphasis was gradually shifted away from issues prioritized by young d/Deaf people, and towards problem-solving to advance the well-being of service providers. Later on, fascinating insights into the resistance that staff felt towards focusing on the views of young d/Deaf people could be gleaned from comments made in their evaluations of the research. For example 'would we as teachers of the hearing impaired have asked more pertinent and relevant questions?' and '[the most interesting thing to emerge was] the inability of students to see [the] true picture of provision as distinct from their own experiences'. It was clear that the service was working under a tremendous strain, and that before staff would look at ways to develop their own effectiveness in meeting the needs identified by the young d/Deaf people, greater involvement of managers in helping staff to identify things they could change would be essential. Local politics were a much more potent force for implementation of change than the experience of young d/Deaf people reflected through the research. It seemed to us that researchers aiming to promote enablement of disabled people through research need to recognize a myriad of constraints which inevitably surround their efforts.

Thinking points

What can you do to ensure that disabled people are involved in both creation and dissemination of research productions? Why is it critical that disabled people themselves disseminate findings from research focusing on their lives? Think about how such a strategy might break down resistance and increase the possibility that research data and recommendations will be taken seriously. What is the trouble with second-hand representation of other people's views? On the other hand, what vulnerabilities are exacerbated if disabled people provide feedback on critical research findings about services which they use? Should (and if so how can) the risks faced by those who operate as the messenger be reduced?

Limiting scope for disempowerment

After the training session we received two letters from the service. One was from the staff development coordinator thanking us for a 'very thought-provoking session', noting that 'the feedback has contained strong feelings!' and commenting that 'people seemed very impressed with your organization of the session'. The second was from one of the post-16 teachers with whom we had planned our input. It was lengthy and expressed unambiguous disappointment 'about what I saw as a missed opportunity'. In a quick dissection of the letter, several points become obvious. The writer intended, perhaps knowingly (certainly authoritatively – 'if I am proved wrong, I will gladly eat my hat'), that the unequal power relationship which exists between service users and service providers should be accentuated through research in ways which render disabled people more vulnerable. The unmistakable message was that the report session should function as a catalyst for misrepresentation and violation of disabled people's experiences. Useful research outcomes were viewed as those which might advance the interests of non-disabled service providers, and the needs of disabled people were considered secondary. All this is made quite clear in two extracts from the letter:

The initial error seemed to me to be the failure to differentiate between what I call genuine and pseudo-issues. . . . What I mean is that the students' perceptions of the educational process may in some cases have been correct and, where based on experience in [our Service], may be seen as cause for concern by our Service. On the other hand their perceptions may for a variety of reasons be incorrect or not applicable to this Service. An example from my experience will illustrate this. Some students complained of poor Careers Guidance. Some from certain backgrounds may have had good cause to complain; any from our Service who complained simply had bad, confused memories. . . . The problem was that your manner of presentation suggested that there was a whole list of issues raised by the report all of which were equally urgent and demanding of attention by our Service, whereas really many were pseudo issues.

And, highlighting a lack of regard for the knowledge and experience of the young disabled people:

I hoped we would be able to initiate some development in areas of the Service where the research had suggested there might be room for improvement, but *only* where staff generally considered the criticisms made in the research were legitimate.

The personal criticism was hard to take and we painstakingly examined our own inadequacies in handling the situation that had developed. Perhaps we should have recognized the reluctance of the staff to relinquish power over planning the day and considered their reasons in greater depth. Their desire to keep control could be seen as understandable as they had credibility to lose or gain through having set up the research in the first place. They had viewed the training session as an opportunity to further their own agenda and not that of either the d/Deaf participants or the wider service. They needed to be seen to be doing a good job with the d/Deaf school leavers. We could have tightened our understanding of these motivations and provided what the post-16 teachers regarded as a more apposite training initiative. But bowing to the aspirations of service providers was not a route which we viewed as likely to be representing the interests of young d/Deaf school leavers, and despite criticisms of our efforts, we felt sanguine about, though shaken by, our attempts to retain a focus on ideas from the school leavers themselves.

Despite increasing reservations we were having about the research with regard to implementation of change, the d/Deaf participants themselves provided a great boost to morale and helped to sustain belief that finding a way of conveying their views was a worthwhile goal. When set-backs made us think of abandoning the project, the young d/Deaf people themselves convinced us that their stories needed telling and their suggestions taking seriously. In addition, the Deaf advisers prompted us to think about ways of maximizing the impact of the research *beyond* the service we were working within, and this finally provided the most profitable route for providing opportunities for personal growth and change.

The Deaf advisers had suggested that the young d/Deaf interviewees could contribute directly to specialist magazines for hearing impaired people. Several of the young d/Deaf people thought that a national magazine for d/Deaf children and their families would reach a relevant readership, and the editors responded enthusiastically to the idea of providing a forum for their views. A number of those who had been interviewed then agreed to produce an article about aspects of their post-school experiences upon which taking part in the research had prompted them to reflect. Photographs were duly taken, each young person wrote an article, and there was a great sense of excitement and achievement when these were published as part of a two page spread on their experiences (National Deaf Children's Society (NDCS) 1993). At last we felt that some progress towards personal empowerment of young d/Deaf people *had* been engendered by their involvement in research, and they felt that their views were wending their way towards an important audience. By relinquishing the notion that we as researchers had to take singular responsibility for disseminating the views of the researched, and responding to d/Deaf people's own ideas about publication options, an avenue was opened up for young d/Deaf school leavers to speak for themselves, to reach an audience of their own choosing and to recognize that they were entitled to have their views taken seriously. We are not so naive as to presume that this evens out the imbalance in the research relationship or gives a particularly wide voice to any participant, but it was a beginning and one that provided an opportunity for those young people to recognize the importance that other people might attach to their views.

In 1995 the reflections of the d/Deaf interviewees were featured again in a national poster campaign promoting careers options for hearing impaired school leavers. This provided further testimony to the value that disabled people's own representative agencies attached to the views of young d/Deaf people, and was in stark contrast to the way in which educational services had deliberately tried to ensure that their views would be marginalized. While we greatly value these outcomes personally, because they were determined and directed by disabled people themselves, we have also had to accept that our research productions were of little value within the professional systems in which our research is accredited.

Tom Shakespeare (1996) has pointed to the lack of fit which can exist between disabled people's own representations of their experience and the articulations which academic researchers are encouraged to make of those same experiences. 'Points of View' items for family friendly magazines, leaflets for campaigns run by voluntary agencies and participation in the development of articles intended to be read in the voices of, and forums encountered by, disabled people themselves, which were the outputs of the project under discussion, may constitute dissemination which can make a difference in the lives

of disabled people and their families. However, within university life such outputs are not afforded the same status as articles in peer reviewed academic
journals likely to be seen primarily by research colleagues (Higher Education
Funding Council 1996). It is fortunate that journals are beginning to appear
which both include, and reach out to, disabled people as well as academic audi-
ences – for example, the newly established international *Journal of Community,
Work and Family*, which attempts to tackle these problems with a more inclusive approach to both authorship and readership.

Notwithstanding the above-mentioned difficulties, a route for maximizing
rights for disabled people within the research process (and hence the resulting
personal and collective benefits) was emerging which we would now have
used from the beginning: that of researching alongside disabled people first,
and involving relevant service providers second. It was clear that young d/Deaf
people had very little experience of having their views taken into account from
comments made by one who wrote 'it feels weird to be in TALK magazine . . .
it's surprising that I'm being asked to feature in it'. The writer then went on to
give in detail 'My message for parents and other people in connection with the
deaf' (NDCS 1993). On reading this we finally realized that our insistence on
a research agenda defined by young d/Deaf people themselves had facilitated
confidence and a greater awareness of personal effectiveness for those who
had taken part. The change of approach to working directly with the young
d/Deaf people felt constructive, clear and much more comfortable and productive than the process of working with professionals.

Getting out

It was tempting to acquiesce to service providers at this point. We had gained
their written permission 'to make any use of the research you see fit', but
enticing as it was to take the report and extract ourselves, we would have
been failing on many counts had we done this. First, we felt accountable to
the participants to try to see things through to a more satisfactory in-service
conclusion. Second, we remained committed to the research findings which
we felt justified service development. Third, the service had approached us
well before the training day on the issue of introducing the Deaf advisers to
the management and post-16 team with a view to developing their possible
involvement with service users. By now however, the post-16 teachers were
open about their reluctance to continue research in connection with us, with
our irksome emphasis on inclusion of d/Deaf people in the process: '[we] did
not realize you were considering the next phase so soon!' They were evidently keen to get us safely out of the way: '[we] feel it best if you contact . . .'.
But we knew that our Deaf advisers valued our link with the post-16 teachers
as a possible way in to the service. They hoped to use this inroad to raise various issues for service development in the local area, and so we persevered,
and set up a meeting which would bring members of the service together with
the Deaf people who had acted as advisers to the project.

It was important to get this meeting right in order to set the newly emerging relationship between the two parties off on a positive start. In line with general good practice for facilitating communication between d/Deaf and hearing people, and the preference of the Deaf individuals taking part, we suggested circulation of an agenda in advance of the meeting. We were immediately in trouble with the service again: 'an agenda – it all sounds so formal!' wrote one of the teachers; 'we would prefer not to have a specified agenda but to keep the meeting as an opportunity for general discussion . . . I hope this meets with [the Deaf advisers'] approval'. An inauspicious start, which we felt did not bode well for the right of disabled people to full access to discussion. Once again, disabled people's views were not being valued.

The meeting turned out to be disastrous. The teacher who had written to say 'I really don't see this [meeting] as needing an agenda or a chair!' afterwards wrote to apologize 'for my burbling attempts at chairing the meeting', saying 'I had not expected that I would be asked to take that role. Had I known, I could have prepared myself.' We privately wondered why a key representative for a service for hearing impaired people would not prepare to facilitate communication in any situation and could not readily understand why support offered by Deaf people invited to the meeting had been turned down. As the meeting had been overtly controlled by representatives of a supposedly specialist service for hearing impaired people, we had been reluctant in our position as visiting researchers, to intervene when it became apparent that no minutes would be taken, though this should be standard practice for easing effective communication and avoiding misunderstandings when d/Deaf and hearing people take part in meetings together. The entire meeting was an uncomfortable affair. The lack of structure, with no chair, no communication rules, one hearing person saying 'John's a good lip-reader' and talking over the interpreter meant that it was a disabling and patronizing experience for the Deaf people and something we were embarrassed to observe.

We were even more dismayed when after the meeting, service providers wrote to dismiss any possible objections, saying 'the whole point of the meeting (at least as far as we were concerned) was that there should not be a "structure" as such – merely an opportunity to exchange views and ideas.' Undoubtedly, anything more substantial had been deliberately avoided. A record of the meeting, for example, could have comprised a vehicle for action and inclusion for the d/Deaf representatives of service users. By now, we were completely discontented with the resistance shown by hearing service providers to the views of d/Deaf service users and their allies. We decided we could no longer work with the service and this was to be the end of our contact. We wrote to the Deaf advisers to offer our independent support for pursuing any of their ideas for service development or further research. Meanwhile the post-16 teachers had told us that they had decided that any subsequent meetings with the Deaf advisers should take place away from the service offices. In their proposal that further meetings should be held elsewhere, 'rather than everyone coming [here]', we observed a thinly veiled attempt, yet again, to resist the rights to inclusion of d/Deaf people; non-d/Deaf service providers were reinforcing their power over d/Deaf people by keeping them away from their territory and structuring subsequent meetings on *their* terms. Some time later we were not surprised when one of the post-16 teachers wrote to say 'I have still not heard anything from [the Deaf advisers]'.

The process of getting out without selling out is a difficult one which researchers at times have to face. It was clear that for us, and the service, the notion of collaborative research to promote empowerment was viewed completely differently. For example, when the Deaf advisers requested a meeting to exchange views and ideas sparked by the research with service providers, they were told in writing that this would be viewed 'purely as an information-giving session'. A letter was sent to us saying:

> [the advisers have been] sent a list of things [the service is] involved with so that [they] can get some idea beforehand. Hopefully we can chat about these in more detail. . . . If [the advisers'] purpose for the meeting is anything other than this, then maybe we should look again at what [they are] suggesting.

There was little prospect of placing control of discussions in the hands of disabled people. There was no notion of reciprocity, or gain for the community of disabled people who were seeking to use the research to facilitate the process of their empowerment. Repeatedly, intensive efforts to dismantle barriers surrounding the evolution of empowerment prospects through research were made in vain. There seemed little sense in pressing on with further joint work.

A project worth doing?

The aftermath of research had certainly created problems, not only for us as researchers, but also for the informants and those service providers who had controlled the research activity. We had all gained different things from the project, some good and some bad. As researchers we had learned many lessons about the limited scope for promoting the rights of disabled users in projects controlled by non-disabled service providers. We had battled to achieve some positive personal outcomes for d/Deaf people who were involved in the study, and learned the hard way that any success in promoting the interests of service users was wholly dependent on developing aims and objectives from their own starting points in the first place. A mixture of caution and naïvety had led us initially to seek out non-disabled service providers as allies in the production of research. Once more, we were finding that the nature of commitment in service-related research is a complex and entangled matter. Those providing services may neither believe nor accept that their obligations involve promoting service users' rights to self-determination.

By the end of the project we had faced the fact that disabled people are their own best allies, and that professionals within relevant support services may well not have the promotion of service users rights at heart. The critical reflection of this project has again been crucial to our learning as researchers. It is through this process that we have come to realize more fully that the business of managing priorities to maximize empowerment of disabled people through research can be satisfactorily managed only if the priorities underlying a project are those of disabled people themselves. To achieve this, non-disabled researchers need to work *first* with those who have direct, personal experience of disablement.

Conclusions

This chapter has brought into focus the issue of power and control in research projects. We went into a context hoping to allow a range of stakeholders their own agenda without realizing the formidable effect of power structures on the way the research could move. We ended this project by concluding that contrary to the research teachings of our respective academic backgrounds, it is *not* necessarily useful for researchers to be neutral or value free. It became impossible at times to keep our own views hidden as we tried to build an inquiry alongside non-disabled service providers when we felt the priorities of disabled service users were being submerged. Thus, at best, our research efforts must have appeared ill thought out and at worst, to be undermining of collaborative inquiry.

What we should have done, with the benefit of hindsight, is to have owned up to our personal commitment to promoting the rights of disabled people through the research. It would have been more productive to dispense with the façade of impartiality which we had tried to hold on to, in order to pacify service providers, even though we knew ourselves to be allied with service users. We could have avoided finding ourselves in a world of subterfuge and evasion by refusing to distance ourselves from the interests of disabled people. By realigning ourselves as co-researchers with disabled people first it might have been possible to openly maximize prospects for empowerment through research. At this point, however, we persuaded ourselves that the experiences recounted in this chapter had been dominated by an unfortunate set of relations and circumstances. After taking stock, we decided that service providers in a different context might perhaps be less preoccupied with political axes to grind, and more willing to engage in rights-based, equality oriented research influenced and led by disabled people.

Thinking points

What strategies can be invoked to ensure that disabled people do not experience alienation from the research process? How can researchers place their methodological expertise in the hands of those who wish to use research as a vehicle in the struggle against personal or collective oppression? And how can the prospect of empowerment through research be presented to disabled people who have not yet considered possibilities for greater self-determination? What mechanisms can researchers put into place which will enable disabled people who are not connected with research institutions to access those institutions and instigate collaborative inquiry? What mechanisms can disability organizations put into place which will enable researchers to respond to their research requirements? How do researchers create alliances with disabled people, and how do disabled people create alliances with researchers? How does your own research activity measure up in relation to these questions?

4

Making commitment: siding with disabled people

Introduction

The chief lesson to be learned from previous chapters is that a research approach which places disabled people at the centre of its processes and analyses is essential. This notion is gaining increasing attention in research (Burton and Kagan 1996; Oliver 1996; Sample 1996) but we discovered through the research efforts documented thus far that unless disabled people are listened to from the earliest inception of a project, opportunities for researchers to respond effectively to their input are restricted. The focal project in this chapter reveals our attempts to bring the rhetoric of listening to disabled people to the forefront of our own disability research practice.

We have found ourselves forced to consider carefully what is involved for listening to be enabling, and have concluded that this depends on several things. Clear exposition of the researcher's role is important. There is a need for clarification of whether researchers are acting as passive listeners, with either no acknowledged political agenda, or one so clearly stated that it is clear how they intend to interpret what they are told, or whether they are operating as active listeners and so will openly engage in debate, declare their own experiences and challenge material which they are unhappy with. Contemplating these issues has presented us with the uncomfortable challenge of relinquishing control and power over research proceedings for which we were professionally accountable. But we found that through taking the risk of acknowledging our own vulnerabilities and letting go of our professional expertise, we actually gained considerably as researchers. In addition, criticisms anticipated from academic peers, of our efforts to research in unconventional ways, turned out not to be worth worrying about because what we lost through shedding professional power and mystique, we regained through enhancing the accessibility and meaning of the research for disabled people, their families and their allies.

In this chapter key issues will be examined with reference to a qualitative interview study designed to look at the experience of d/Deaf children and their families. As in the research with young d/Deaf people discussed in Chapter 3, our aim was to place informants plainly in charge when determining research topics. In contrast with previous projects, however, where we had been working as external agents of change, we realized that we now needed to work from a different position.

An opportunity arose within a service we were working for, to try conducting research from an insider perspective. There would be obvious links to 'action research' as a mode of self-reflective inquiry which encourages practitioners to become researchers of their own practice in order to enhance the quality of service for themselves and for service users (McNiff 1988; Whyte 1991). We had affirmed our commitment to respecting service users' rights to have their views known and taken seriously and we hoped, as internal research agents, that there would be real potential for bringing about broad changes of attitude and practice based on any research findings. But doubts about our personal efficacy quickly began to creep in when uncovering the experience of service users proved controversial and unsettling to colleagues for whom the research findings would have most relevance.

When, as within-service researchers, we identified problems with our own service we could not be satisfied simply with relaying information in the hope of stimulating change. If we did not agitate for change, then we ourselves were inescapably part of the problem. When we did agitate for change, we both created, and experienced, serious problems in the workplace. The enormity of the waves which can be created through within-service research need to be fully recognized: once researchers make their commitments known many social and political consequences follow (Homan 1991: 157). In our own case, refusal to keep quiet about the limitations of the service which our research was uncovering resulted in such turbulence that we had no alternative but to resign from our posts.

The chapter will show how even as within-service researchers, phenomenal resistance can be encountered towards activities which might stimulate implementation of change based on the priorities of service users. Our own experience has led us to become more cautious about service-based research and development, and move increasingly towards researching directly with disabled people in the wider context of their lives, rather than in the narrow context of their experiences of particular services. We did have reservations about this change because it seemed inevitable that the practical and policy implications of research would be even more limited if research was conducted without direct service links. In the end we chose to operate from yet another new 'researcher position', completely severing links with relevant services and professionals. The relative merits of 'insider' vs. 'outsider' research for influencing service delivery are discussed in this chapter in order to emphasize the necessity for disabled people's active participation in constructing research which informs the services they encounter.

In this chapter we aim to

- explore in some depth the difficulties of being within-service researchers, notably the dangers therein of perpetuating established patterns of oppression
- focus on risk taking by, and coping strategies for, researchers when control over critical aspects of project design, processes of analysis and dissemination is handed over to service users
- illustrate how relinquishing researcher control enhances the meaning and utility of data
- comment on the changing character of research when disabled people are active participants in every aspect of the processes of inquiry.

The project described in this chapter considered the experiences of having a d/Deaf child in the family (Beazley and Moore 1995).

Context and getting started

We were working for a service which provided support for families of young preschool children diagnosed as being deaf. The service was unusual in that it was not organized by a local authority but based at an academic institution involved in educating professionals at graduate and postgraduate level with provision through a range of clinics for assessment and ongoing management of hearing impairment. Clinics provided students with a chance to observe others working and also to develop their own skills. Families were encouraged to view the service as part of a centre of excellence where new and interesting suggestions and approaches might be found for them and their child.

The service was run very much along lines of the medical model of disability with a heavy emphasis on the individual needs of children with hearing impairment for adapting to a hearing world. As in many long-established services and institutions, a clearly defined hierarchy existed among the staff and positions were secured in the pecking order through various trappings of professionalism, such as international notoriety and publications in highly revered academic journals might afford. The medical setting, together with a climate of individual self-interest provided a strange context in which to commence research taking the social model of disability as its starting point, but as such, it did comprise a context which was arguably crying out for greater acknowledgement of the social construction of disablement. We were provided with funding by the university to develop research relating to the family support which we were involved in providing, and thus led to believe not only that change was possible, but also desired, by those in positions of power. It seemed we occupied a much stronger position as within-service researchers than in previous research endeavours where we had operated as unfunded outsiders.

One condition was imposed upon our receipt of funding for the research project, and this was that we would involve two nominated service providers as co-researchers. The research team subsequently comprised ourselves – a lecturer in psychology and a speech and language therapist – plus our peers, the two co-researchers, from backgrounds in teaching and audiology, both of whom were involved in providing the family support service. With this range of expertise within the team we thought that the project would offer considerable prospects for both within-service and beyond-service development. We were, however, all non-disabled researchers and yet again about to discover that disabled people and their representatives are habitually denied access to the research process which, as we have already argued, ultimately leads to research outcomes from which they are unable to profit. By the time of writing now, both from our own extensive experiences and our knowledge of other research accounts, we are informed enough to believe that for many researchers, denying disabled people and their representatives access to research processes is deliberate and strategic rather than accidental and of little significance.

Thinking points

How well do you know the setting for your research as an internal agent? How well do you know the motivations and preoccupations of your co-researchers? Are there any obstacles which might impede the progress of research within your research team? It is worth thinking through what these might be before starting the project. Think about strategies for dealing with obstacles either prior to their occurrence or as they arise. For example, if you are worried about 'X's attitude to involving disabled people in the project', you might consider (a) establishing a forum for discussing your different perspectives, (b) developing some ground rules to ensure representation of disabled people's views, (c) identifying your line manager and setting up a structure for keeping them informed of any differences within the team and how they are resolving. Think before you start about any mechanisms you can put in place to maintain relationships within the research team when there are conflicting personal and political agendas. Such planning could well turn out to be a lifeline, even if at the beginning of your project you feel quite certain that difficulties are unlikely to arise.

Evolving a within-service research project

The process of coming up with a research project was chiefly the responsibility of the two of us in receipt of research funding, who were required to work up a project in collaboration with two other colleagues, who were obliged to engage in these research activities as part of their regular jobs. The four of us together decided to set up an exploratory research project during which we would meet a number of families using the service and discover their views on parenting a d/Deaf child, with particular reference to their experiences of professionals and our own service.

The team met weekly to review progress in aspects of research design; differences of opinion about the nature of the research enterprise quickly began to be uncovered. For instance, there was some debate about research needing to contain 'real' measures not 'just' users' views. The appropriateness of involving d/Deaf adults, and/or parent users of the service in the research team, proved to be a source of contention and prompted much stalling. There was constant pressure from one member of the team to include so-called 'objective measures' of audiological assessment in the inquiry, which seemed to stem from the medical ethos of the organization as a whole with its historic and evangelical preference for quantitative research.

Once again, we faced resistance to two aspects of research which were important to us; first, possibilities for embracing some prospect for promoting the rights of service users were being curtailed, and second, attempts to explore the social origins of disablement were being suppressed. Given that time for the project was limited, we had to compromise as individuals within a team. Instead of holding out for a project that was wholly determined by service users themselves, it was settled that two of us would be satisfied if the project included an open-ended qualitative component enabling parents to put forward their own views and ideas about family life with a d/Deaf child and experiences of support. The other two agreed to go ahead if the project could additionally pursue measures of audiological assessment.

The process of setting up within-service evaluative research is fraught with potential difficulties. The threat of watering down personal convictions about the nature of research becomes particularly virulent when trying to maintain positive relations with co-researchers who are colleagues in a variety of contexts. By the time of carrying out this project we had developed an almost reverent respect for maintaining good interpersonal relationships within research, and we were at this stage doing everything we could by way of bringing friendly overtures to meetings, arranging evenings with pizzas so that we could 'get to know each other better' and so on, all in the spirit of creating and helping to maintain positive and comfortable working relationships. There is a fine line to negotiate, however, when trying to balance the social function of efforts to listen and be supportive to one's colleagues, with the need to function as a productive and effective working research team.

Who knows what?

Within the time scheduled for project completion we could not hope to meet all the families who used the service and so needed to find a way of deciding which families to involve. The two team members connected full-time with running the service began to nominate those whom they thought could cope with participation, and immediately we had run into the old problem of researchers restricting access for disabled people and their representatives to take part in research. Open access could have been arranged easily with all potential families being offered the opportunity to participate, even if we might have to explain that not everyone approached could be interviewed in the initial stages. Families could themselves have been asked for suggestions of how we could select families if there were too many to meet. Those who could not be interviewed could have been invited to send in some of their experiences on audio or video tape or in written form if they wished. Alternatively, group discussions could have been organized in the first instance. None of this happened, however, as our colleagues were insistent that some families were not suitable for inclusion.

Sometimes reasons for excluding a family from the research were made specific, for example, participation would be 'too much to expect' of families who had recently received the diagnosis of their child's hearing impairment or who had other worries at home. However, when professionals make decisions about who to 'protect' from research, this has the effect of diminishing other people's rights and of excluding people who could have made the decision for themselves about whether or not they wished to share their experiences with others. Other reasons for excluding certain families were not so explicit, but the politics of relations with local services was intimated to be another good reason for exclusion, as was competition for the 'rights to research subjects' within the organization. The critical factor to note at this point however, is that in the interests of retaining harmony within our own service, the two of us, who should by now have known much better, did agree to compromise over which families would be invited to join in with the research.

Emergence of misgivings

By now, even though the two of us looking back at this project were busily glossing over differences of opinion among the four members of the research team, it had become evident that divisions existed. We two had set ourselves up as wanting to promote the interests of service users, whereas our two colleagues were committed to promoting only those interests of service users which suited their agenda as service providers. This split was openly acknowledged, although in order for it to be so, we found ourselves positioned as the two members of the team who were least mindful of what issues for service providers were. Thus our efforts to position ourselves as the allies of service users resulted in our professional credibility being quietly undermined. We thought that we could accept this if investing our colleagues with a superior sense of their own expertise was a prerequisite for moving the project further forward. This amounted, however, to the furthering of oppression for service users whose well-being was being further 'owned' by researchers closely aligned with the medical model of understanding disability issues.

Our next move towards evening out medical model vs. social model approaches to our inquiry was to suggest that interviews should be conducted by interviewers working in interchangeable pairs. Ostensibly this was intended to ensure some balance and consistency in interviewing approach and to develop greater confidence in working together as a team. In addition, interviewing in pairs would engineer some equity in the way in which the research would be presented to the families. Such an arrangement was bound to be difficult, because it entailed deliberate contrivance of pairs in which the two interviewers each knew themselves to be pursuing research objectives in quite different ways. This was a problem that we tried to acknowledge openly, and to frame not only as beneficial in the interests of research integrity, but also as providing opportunities for professional development for all four team members. Just as it seemed we could go ahead and meet the families, one of the team retracted and refused to conduct interviews with the one of us with whom she felt her personal and theoretical views were most diametrically opposed.

When a group of colleagues are trying to work together on within-service research, hostility within the team is undesirable. The team members have each to work alongside each other on other professional tasks beyond the research, and all concerned are motivated to be seen to be doing their own tasks well. If one person refuses to research alongside another, clearly an unacceptable level of antagonism is introduced and the rejected colleague feels insecure. In our situation, this person was rendered particularly vulnerable because, in our efforts to keep the needs of service users uppermost in the research and, at the same time, retain harmonious working relations, we had previously permitted our colleague to undermine some of our professional credibility. In effect, we had been saying to our co-researchers 'we are prepared to accept that you best know the concerns of service providers, so we will concentrate on the concerns of service users'; our motive here was to ensure consideration of the service users' agenda, but this made it possible for our co-researchers to deprecate our understanding of issues for professionals. Consequently, when our co-researchers wished to assert their preference for research which made no reference to the rights of service users it was easy to exploit the risk we had taken which had serious consequences for our professional credibility.

This pattern of events is likely to be characteristic of what happens in the context of much within-service research. Undoubtedly, the presence of disabled adults, and/or parents of d/Deaf children, within the project team would have made an enormous difference. The inclusion of disabled people and their representative family members would have thrown into sharp relief questions about the locus of expertise, and helped to ensure that the focus of research activity remained firmly with the interests of the user group rather than the concerns of researchers. However, we had allowed two members of our team to resist the inclusion of disabled people and their family representatives.

The refusal of our colleagues to accept that disabled people and their representative family members could contribute appropriate (and in our view essential) expertise, is typical of the cultural climate in agencies with strong medical links where a great deal is invested in making sure professional expertise is rarefied. Professionals are deemed to know best, and this myth is protected by the notion that disabled people and their representatives lack appropriate 'objectivity' and must necessarily remain at a distance from explorations of disability issues. We had discovered that it is not enough for non-disabled researchers to position themselves as allies of disabled people in research endeavours; we needed disabled people to be *our* allies if there was to be any prospect of a project which could resist characteristic medical system oppression.

It may appear that many difficulties in executing this research project stemmed from problems to do with personalities in the team. What we hope to have exposed is a rather more disturbing and substantial theoretical under-side to differences in the way in which disability researchers approach their investigations. In our team, the origins of difference could be traced back to investment in medical vs. social understandings of disability. The most 'medical model' person refused to work alongside the most 'social model' person, with the intention of preventing medical model explanations being diluted by reference to social phenomena.

The underlying problem here was that any social explanations for research findings would be discounted. Whereas three of the team were happy to accept divergent perspectives and pool understandings of the origins of dis-ablement in the interests of providing the strongest possible explanation of the families' experiences, the dissenting team member was keen to uphold her personal theoretical viewpoint and did not wish to evaluate her own prac-tice. She preferred to work with colleagues united in the belief that it is non-disabled professionals, and *not* people with impairments and/or their family members, who best know the business of disabled people's lives.

All of this meant that we now had a tangible split. Only the presence of dis-abled people and/or their representative family members could have helped to avoid the conflicts rising from personal and academic differences that were proving so detrimental to the study. The unique insight that disabled people themselves can offer into the limitations of medical explanations of their experience would have gone a long way towards ensuring social perspectives were less easily undermined, even in the climate of historic veneration for medical approaches in which we were operating.

Despite concerted effort, there were evidently difficulties within our research team and so the four of us decided, in the interests of retaining a suf-ficiently tight focus, to try and clarify our roles and relations. We needed to avoid getting side-tracked into questions of 'who wouldn't tolerate such a viewpoint' or 'who wouldn't work with who', and to keep discussions firmly fixed on completing a profitable piece of research. Several actions were taken to formalize our activities, included specifying time of start and finish times for meetings, circulating agenda items in advance and building in a specific slot for raising non-research issues, for which we would organize another meeting. We rotated chairing responsibilities for each session with a view to ensuring balance and shared responsibility for getting tasks done. However, these tactics served only to aggravate matters and polarize differences. One of the team members now seemed committed to ending the entire project and to this end either monopolized the agenda or failed to attend meetings, so that progress was thwarted.

Frustration, worry and misunderstandings continued to escalate and we, as the two funded researchers, became anxious that we were not going to meet our job requirements. At this point we decided to speak to our line manager and so began the short and unpleasant part of our careers which culminated in our resignations. It seems unlikely that an individual non-disabled team member would have resisted active involvement of disabled people and their families in the management and design of the project with such unremitting insistence if representatives of the service user group had been in a position to witness such motivations and behaviour through participation in research meetings.

Our line manager encouraged us to begin interviews with families but we quickly found that they had discerned the division that had occurred and were fearful that participating in the project would jeopardize their entitlement to service provision. One mother we tried to arrange to interview was confused to hear from us; we were dismayed when she named our dissenting team member as having explicitly advised that it would be best for her and her child if she did not talk to us. We interpreted this as bullying. We were becoming increasingly concerned at the oppressive nature of various practices that we were observing and fearful that our very association with such domination meant that we were part of its perpetuation. We went back again to talk to our line manager as it was now becoming imperative, for both personal and professional reasons, to distance our own research activities from those of other colleagues.

Risk taking

The research was being hindered by immovable reverence for the medical model of disability within the team, and for the power which investment in medical model explanations affords (at least superficially) to non-disabled professionals. We were not prepared to fortify the power of professionals by conducting a project aimed at sustaining the myth that professionals know best what service users need. Although our reflections may seem rather self-important and pretentious, we were motivated mainly through fear of being disowned by our disabled friends, fellow researchers and other allies who might ask us to clarify our reasons for proceeding without adequate inclusion of disabled people's own voices. In view of the continuing problems, we approached our line manager yet again for ideas about how best to proceed.

This is where we began to detect that the process of gathering data was becoming an intensely political one. Reasons for obstruction were a matter of conjecture, but our worst suspicions were quickly confirmed when we were told that the main priority behind our receipt of research funding was for the centre's publication record to be improved. We had been recruited because we were known locally for our ability to remain reasonably unruffled in tricky research situations, and for willingness to operate as conciliators in the face of interpersonal disharmony. The intention was that we might be able to carry a research team and help to ensure that names of colleagues would appear on a respectable number of publications for the year. At least, these are our own self-defensive suppositions, supported by the frank explanations that we were given when we sought to clarify our concerns and move the project on.

We had to accept new possibilities about the intentions behind our research funding. It was openly established that the project was funded for the particular purpose of improving the academic profile of the service. It seemed plain that improvement to services for d/Deaf children and their families within the centre was not the principal hoped-for outcome. We had taken the risk of entering into within-service action research, knowing that this would demand a considerable degree of self-exposure and would not necessarily be a cosy or self-affirming activity, because we had genuinely believed support to be on offer for the collection of data which would advance empowerment of service users. We had discovered, to the contrary, that empowerment prospects generated by the research were to be reserved for service providers. *Dis*empowerment of disabled people was not considered, as the paramount need was for the service to appear productive, even if its productions were (as we saw it) to damage and undermine the interests of disabled service users.

Our assumption that the research funders had a prime interest in the experience of service users was rudely dispelled. Personal, practical and policy relevances for disabled people were turning out to be immaterial. Resistance to involvement of service users in the project team had been propped up by the management's desire to primarily promote the interests of the centre through adding up research points. Vexing negotiations over inclusion of service users within the research team, which had effectively stalled operationalization of the project, could not be properly dealt with because the departmental line was to elevate interests of the service and by default to do so over and above those of service users. Disempowering research which produced measures and findings that families with d/Deaf children did not themselves prioritize was regarded as acceptable, being easy to execute and easy to get published in sufficiently obscure academic journals. Research and promotion of the rights of participants within it were regarded as all very well, but if researchers were not inclined to respond to the interests of service users, then the empowerment dimension was framed as being, and accepted by management to be, more trouble than it was worth.

To continue with the project once we had come to understand these motivations would have reinforced disablement. Yet again we were up against the structural domination of the medical model and its institutions in disabled people's lives. Our intention to conduct research which might *enable* d/Deaf children and their families was frustrated by the need to retain power by service providers. Our eventual decision to resign because we were unable to oppose the stranglehold of the medical model climate illustrates something of the power of cultural creed within the organization we were working in.

Thinking points

At this juncture it is worth considering again the workings of your own research team. In all working groups there are individuals competing for influence or resources; there are differences of opinions and of values, conflicts of priorities and of goals. What do you know about the positions and motivations of those in your own team? How are the workings of your team influenced by the inclusion or exclusion of any disabled members? On disability research projects conducted exclusively by non-disabled researchers, we have encountered a myriad of general, deleterious effects to do with power structures and interpersonal processes within such groups. Why is it likely that in research teams comprising both disabled and non-disabled researchers, more effective action will be possible for transcending ideological domination? What implications does the 'disabled/non-disabled researcher constitution' of your team have for your research outcomes?

Facing up to oppression in research

Once the working research group had become split, we risked being drawn further into the 'politics' of the organization, expending most of our energy on this and less on the research task. As it became evident that we could not progress with the research agenda within the specified group, we obtained permission to run the project independently. Immediately, new barriers then began to be erected, not only against us, but also against the line manager who agreed to continuation of the work, with the now former team members openly attempting to oppose the study. Other researchers will recognize the destructive and demoralizing repercussions of such episodes. Memos were going to and fro in endeavours to stop the research, but we had full approval from the head of department and so tried to get on with the job of mounting a project which we continued to hope would provide tangible benefit for d/Deaf children and their families who used the service. Then we received the following memo from a member of staff who had no formal involvement with our activities whatsoever:

> I understand that you are planning to carry out research involving parents of children attending these clinics. If this is so then where children are the responsibility of either Dr R or myself then we would expect to be consulted before this research is carried out. I suggest that you let us have a copy of your protocol and discuss it with us before you take any steps such as contacting the parents about your research.

This presumed ownership of sole access rights to a group of people exemplifies disempowerment and infringement of individual rights in the extreme. Doubtless this occurs in many other contexts where the medical model presides and non-disabled professionals permit themselves to believe that they are experts and the rightful managers of the lives of disabled service users and their families. Our view was that service *users* had the greatest entitlement to *'expect to be consulted before this research is carried out'*. The suggestion that the approval of service providers must be ascertained before service users could be invited to make their views known was clearly intended primarily to protect the interests of professionals. Our prime object for the research, however, was to urge insight into the perspective of disabled people and their families, in order to prompt change which they themselves prioritized.

The project was by now infused with considerable tension. The only course was to re-route the research plans. At this point, in order to have a way of looking at relevant issues in a more enabling perspective, with disabled people and their families positioned as experts, and non-disabled professionals prevented from shoring up the myth that they know best, we decided we would have to withdraw from all connections with the centre. We realized that we would be able to pursue the project to much greater effect, with greatly reduced personal costs and without perpetuating such oppressive practices, if we were no longer part of the organization and hence, being less than half way through the funded period, we tendered our resignation. This was not a glamorous or powerful statement but an action arising out of despair, unending anxiety and misery. Our resignations initially created isolation for us and frustration because a sense of professionalism bound us to be cautious about how we explained our actions to others. Our disabled allies, and contacts with those in representative agencies, provided a bridge, enabling us to know that other people would realize that the breakdown was not entirely our fault. But we experienced considerable awkwardness due to not being able to share the full details of what had led us to such drastic departures and we were not resistant to the ensuing personal embarrassment and pain. We had endeavoured to find allies within the system and to try to stay in, but this had proved impossible.

We were later to realize that our greatest allies were each other. The role of friendship in research relations has been identified as a crucial element of support by other writers (Miller 1990; A. Edwards and Talbot 1994). Mutual trust and comfortable acceptance of value positions have now become the essential ingredient for making sensible headway with any project. There is, of course, a danger of being over-romantic about this. The cultivation of friendship, and especially of critical friendships, which provide scope for open and honest dialogue between researchers is costly in terms of time, emotionality, thought and other relationships. But in such turbulent research environs as under discussion here, where we were driven actually to give up research funding since we believed it had only ever been intended to reinforce disablement and oppression, value placed on friendship is inestimable. It was mainly the pursuit of continuing friendship that enabled us to set about contacting families with d/Deaf children through their representative agencies from our new position as unattached researchers, to pick ourselves up, and think about starting again.

We felt humiliated withdrawing not only from our research commitments, but also from every aspect of our professional involvement with the family support service, and from teaching within this particular university. Our line manager brought in a university dean to persuade us to reconsider, but the climate remained firmly rooted in medical model ideology and consequently unfavourable to research being anything other than oppressive of disabled people. We shrank from straining our relations with disabled people and their representative organizations by conducting research as if our professional qualifications and publications counted for more than their experience, but taking this stance had cost us our salaries and much more besides.

It will be obvious that this project was riddled with problems that should have been avoided, and many questions that should have been reformulated. It had run the risk of becoming incoherent and incomplete, because disabled people and their families had not been involved from the outset. We were ultimately not prepared to accept the risk of incompletion, however, and set about making direct contact with the major national representative agencies of d/Deaf children and their families to elicit their views on research relating to family support. We talked to people at the National Deaf Children's Society who showed interest in developing research and agreed to convene a small committee with ourselves and two parents of d/Deaf children, one hearing and one Deaf to oversee research development.

Changing research relations

By working collaboratively with parent representatives of the National Deaf Children's Society, and following through our original commitment to placing the experience of d/Deaf people and their families in the centre of the frame, we were finally able to develop methodological strategies which would properly investigate their experiences. Not only this, but also we were able to build in strategies for encouraging personal development for those taking part in the project which an anonymous reviewer of our research proposals regard as 'operationalization of emancipatory research [which] is more advanced than any other disability research of which I am currently aware'. The nature of the eventual study, together with a full discussion of data and findings, is fully documented in the book *Deaf Children, their Families and Professionals: Dismantling Barriers* (Beazley and Moore 1995). Confirmation that the research succeeded in its objective of uncovering and disseminating what families with d/Deaf children see as their own needs, rather than what hearing people think d/Deaf children and their families need, came from evaluations made by the families:

> finally someone is listening to what has happened to parents and how they feel – not how other people think we should

[the research] shows that [families] are not alone, deaf children are normal, they'll get through and there's help if wanted

thank you for taking the time to listen to our story, and congratulations on producing a book which is both moving and enlightening.

Conclusions

Successful outcomes were possible only once we had severed links with non-disabled professional research peers and invested all our energies in collaboration with families and agencies representing d/Deaf children. We had discovered, through the use of a critically reflective approach, that the key to meaningful disability research with relevant and practical outcomes lies in relinquishing researcher control over a project and in maximizing efforts to equalize relations between the researcher and the researched. The most important lesson we had learned was to recognize what is in the researcher's power, and what is not. As non-disabled researchers we had to take seriously the worthlessness of attempts to research into disabled people's lives without a mandate from, and inclusion of, disabled people in every stage of a project, right from the earliest dawning of ideas, through research design to dissemination and then to decisions about what to research next.

The next project we conducted sought to investigate the experience of disabled parents (Maelzer *et al.* 1998). Our whole approach was altered, and the inspiration for this study came from a disabled mother who had achieved substantial personal recognition for transforming the rights of disabled people to be parents (Maelzer 1991: 10–14). Only because we cut off links with specific services and worked from the beginning with a disabled parent as a member of our team have we begun to succeed in the establishment of research which genuinely involves, is determined by, and so more adequately uncovers, disabled people's experiences. By changing the relations between researchers and disabled people at grass-roots level within our research team, we hope that we are beginning to evolve a more emancipatory research dimension.

Thinking points

Consider your own position as actual or potential researcher within an organization by taking a large sheet of paper and drawing a circle inside to represent the role you might, or do, occupy at work. Label this with your name and work title. Then draw in smaller peripheral circles to represent *all* the significant others in your role network and indicating their names and roles. Make a chart putting on the left all the roles that make demands on your role. Then, under columns alongside, consider 'their expectations of me', 'my expectations of them'; 'possible conflict areas'; 'possible ways of overcoming potential areas of conflict'. Who are your allies? Why is your position for meaningful disability research strengthened if you can nominate both disabled and non-disabled peers? If your network does not include disabled and non-disabled people, how can you make contacts to fill the gaps?

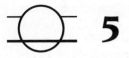 **5**

Uncertain commitment: the interests of children

Introduction

This chapter is structured differently from others because in it we review research principles in relation to a number of projects. Previously we have focused on difficulties which beset a specific piece of work; in this chapter several research activities are returned to in order to emphasize the breadth of concerns which occupy disability researchers whose inquiries involve children. The issues to be discussed in this chapter are often true of children generally, but we argue that they are exacerbated when it comes to disabled children.

Central to questions about children as the focus of research is an understanding of the social construction of childhood. Children's lives cannot be removed from the historical and sociopolitical conditions which inform the agendas and assumptions of researchers, or from appeals to biology and evolution which are invoked for a variety of (often multiple and contradictory) purposes to suit the preferred positions of each individual researcher. Hence, it is important to recognize, for example, that in the UK, notions of 'children', 'childhood' and 'childish' have been long established through a clear separation of authority and status between children and adults, and related cultural assumptions are fundamentally woven into research on disabled children's lives. The powerful role of the separation of children from the division of labour and their non-productive position have also been central to this process. Outcomes include a culture of dependency and an underestimation of children's abilities and possibilities. Notions of childhood and dependency are often entwined in ways which furnish researchers with particular anxieties if they wish to avoid recycling negative images of disability. We hope that placing these problems in the reader's mind, through attempting to identify and review their influences on our own work, will help to guard against indiscriminate application of general research ethics and codes of practice in disability research which involves children.

We wish to urge caution here because, as other writers have noted, research connected with children's lives often turns out to be a route for pathologization of children and of childhood (Burman 1994; Billington 1996). When the focus is on disabled children, then the need to resist this complication is acute. We have major reservations about diverse ways in which our own projects may pathologize children and aim in this chapter to give a flavour of the complexities involved. As already implied, definitions of children and childhood pitch disability researchers into deceptively convoluted territory, and we sketch out some of the quandaries we have come up against. In addition, a host of specific practical and ethical considerations, notably for gaining permissions, establishing confidentiality, handling vulnerability and dealing with disclosure when working with disabled children, compound the difficulties of inquiry. Children's rights are a continual source of worry for those engaging them in research and merit some examination as well (Moore *et al.* 1996). Finally, links between disabled children's research and questions of economics may necessitate some uncomfortable compromises which seem especially relevant to this chapter.

As usual, we wish to urge some redress of the difficulties we describe, rather than just reproduce them.

The chapter aims to

- illustrate ways in which disability research may pathologize children
- examine some of the routine practices and predicaments which concern disability researchers seeking to access children's lives
- promote commitment to warding off some of the injustices which are often recycled both within, and by, research concerning disabled children.

Focal projects

Much of the ensuing discussion relates to studies examined in other chapters; we shall also refer to two further projects. The first of these is work in progress, which explores the experiences of families where parents are the primary providers of care for adult sons and daughters who have learning difficulties (Skelton *et al.* 1997). This study aims to make known the views of learning disabled people (Beazley *et al.* 1998), and their parents (Moore *et al.* 1998) on family life and lifestyle choices. Focus is on developing practical initiatives for enabling learning disabled people and older caregivers to manage transitions in later life, and on developing user-led models of practice.

We shall also discuss a recent project assembling children's reflections on family life (Moore *et al.* 1996). This study had several aims. First, to place children's views firmly at the front of thinking about family friendly policies and practices; second, to illustrate the variety of guises in which children find themselves experiencing family life; third, to provide practical insights for families and professionals based on what children say about the tenor of contemporary family life; and finally, to set an agenda for future child-led discussions. Contributions of relevance to this chapter are from children who had personal experience of impairment within their families, some having learning or physical impairments themselves, or (and sometimes also) having disabled parents, siblings, grandparents or aunts and uncles.

Getting started

In the context of this chapter, 'getting started' refers to deciding that a project will examine aspects of disabled children's lives, and to defining of whom the target child population will consist. These points are often insufficiently scrutinized. As soon as the decision is made to focus on disabled children the risk of pathologizing children with impairments comes to the fore. Arguably, the intention to classify a child as disabled launches the pathologization process, but in order to operationalize a project, we do, of course, need to select children for study. This means that researchers immediately find themselves involved in both labelling and categorizing children, and in rekindling debates about inclusion vs. exclusion, through the processes of selection. Quite clearly these problems characterize our own research.

In the past, we have studied 'hearing impaired children' or 'young d/Deaf people' as focal research populations. We are currently occupied with the experiences of sons and daughters 'with learning difficulties' who live with their parents. All of these studies epitomize the problems mentioned above. While our research questions may be seeking social understanding of the origins of disablement, the projects are oriented in ways which position the nature of impairment almost as if it could be thought of as a dependent variable. Pathologization of children with impairments is reaffirmed through specification of the nature of impairment because the locus of interest consequently falls only partially upon the nature and consequences of the world in which children find themselves. Wherever researchers are interested as we are, in for example, 'the social development of *hearing impaired* children', or 'how services meet the needs of *d/Deaf* school leavers', the problem of objectifying impairment reasserts itself. Research reported elsewhere in this book provides further illustration in respect of this quandary.

The primary focus of research reported in Chapter 2 was – not withstanding recognition of educational context and communication environments – on pupils rendered exotic because the researcher has grouped the children according to impairment. d/Deaf children were problematized and their non-deaf peers assumed the status of a normative group for comparative purposes. Thus, in the reported piece of research, hearing impaired children were positioned as those in need of sorting out. In writing up, researchers can always attempt to resist the most crude ramifications of this problem through judicious presentation of arguments, but such efforts are quite transparent in studies where statistical data have been constituted in terms of information about one population constituting a 'norm' against which to evaluate information relating to a 'significantly different' group.

The ideology of 'normality' is highly questionable; positioning hearing children as members of the 'normal' group makes no more sense than assuming that hearing impaired children are deviant. Hearing children in our research, included in the supposedly 'normal' group for the purposes of comparison with their d/Deaf peers, were not themselves comparable for many different reasons, such as belonging to split or reconstituted families, being members of minority language groups, having multiple commitments, and so on. Many researchers are caught up in reproducing this problem, which also applies to research with disabled adults, for example: 'Acquisition of speech, pre- and post-cochlear implantation: longitudinal studies of a congenitally deaf infant' (Robinshaw 1996); 'Speech error patterns in Cantonese-speaking children with cleft palate' (Stokes and Whitehill 1996); 'Making leisure provision for people with profound learning and multiple disabilities' (Hogg and Cavet 1995). The crucial issue is how do we more appropriately identify and define our research populations? New approaches are urgently required if disability research is to challenge the impairment-led policy and practice of health, welfare and educational institutions. There are difficulties for disability researchers trying to conduct a passage through these concerns, but ways of handling them must be found. There is obviously some obligation to begin contesting the pursuit of normality in the framing of research questions; by accepting responsibility for facing up to, and being explicit about, the reasons why research questions are conceptualized as they are, researchers might start to resist pathologizing disabled children.

Billington (1996) discusses a choice that professionals often need to make between 'constantly reworking' definitions of the 'normal' child, and resisting those definitions because they are fundamentally oppressive. Following Billington's argument we find the same choice befalls researchers identifying disabled children for inclusion in their projects. Researchers will need to decide whether to accept prevailing impairment-led definitions of the child, whether to propose their own definitions, or whether to dispense with impairment as a referent entirely. These decisions need to be openly acknowledged. But since, as always, research is undertaken within the context of institutional and interpersonal conditions and relations, questions of power and control are crucial factors to be engaged with. Whose voice is heard, and whose definition counts, are fundamental concerns and particularly formidable in relation to providing scope for children to define themselves.

Thinking points

What are the implications of grouping children according to impairment within an investigation? How can research questions be framed to avoid the pathologization of children? What alternative ways of organizing participants might lessen allusion to medical models of disability? Where the research topic is specifically impairment linked, is it still possible to look at social phenomena and thus pursue social understandings of a child's experience, behaviour or development? How can you argue

> that research funding and research projects should not be impairment led? What positive contributions can children make towards defining their own status and rights within research?

Definitions of childhood

Following on from problems with definitions and the ideology of normality, we find researchers are confronted with equally vexing definitions of who is a child and what constitutes a childhood. Definitions of the child and of the state of childhood are, inescapably, socially, politically and culturally ascribed (Bradley 1989; Burman 1994). The concept of childhood is laden with meanings, relating most obviously to age, but also to status, generation, occupation, responsibilities and so on. While children, as individuals and as a group, are rendered vulnerable by research classifications, disabled children are particularly likely to be affected by the promotion of injustices through uncertainties surrounding definition of their status.

Most developmental theorists deal with childhood as a maturational process, but this approach quickly proves inadequate in the field of disability studies. Maelzer (1995) writes from personal experience about the oppressive nature of analogies often drawn between a disabled adult's life and that of a baby who is dependent upon another individual for physical, social and emotional support. For non-disabled babies, infant status ends as they become physically independent and assert their rights to privacy and control over their own lives. However, Maelzer (1995) argues, many disabled people are physically and often socially and emotionally dependent on people around them throughout their lives and this can lead to continued application of the labels of infancy, with associated denial of personal power and unwarranted levels of control over disabled people's lives. Some examples from our work involving learning disabled adults show these analogies in operation and confirm that relations between the categories of childhood and adulthood are not clear cut: they pose a perennial problem in disability research:

Mother discussing son in his late 30s:
> I mean it would be somewhere for them to go . . . and there would be other handicapped children as well.

Mother and father describing daughter aged 52:
> *Father*: you see we still look on her as a . . .
> *Mother*: a teenager
> *Father*: a baby type thing
>
> *Father*: she's still a baby, and just a child to be looked after because she's not really capable of looking after herself.

Mother on 31-year-old son:
> he's *not* a 31-year-old . . . you can't treat him like a 31-year-old. If he

was a 31-year-old he'd be out there earning two hundred, three hundred pounds a week.

Mother of her 44-year-old daughter:
   they [social services] don't believe that there should be more than six of these, sort of . . . kids I call them, in one place.

(Skelton *et al.* forthcoming)

The main emphasis in these quotations is on social role, rather than chronological age as a determinant of child or adult identity. Researchers have recently begun to investigate previous neglect of disabled children's own voices in research and literature (T. Shakespeare 1997), but there has been relatively little attempt to clarify what is meant by the concept of childhood in this context, and hence definitions of 'the child' remain ambiguous.

Definitions of maturity and access to various rights and responsibilities have varied greatly over the centuries and over different contexts and cultures. In the UK, for example, the term 'child', as defined for the purposes of the 1989 Children Act, means 'a person of less than 18 years of age' (Smith 1994: 2). In these terms, none of the people described in the quotations from our older caregiver interviewees can be regarded as children, but in terms of reference which are meaningful to their parents, they cannot sensibly be positioned as adults either.

This ambiguity presents our research team with considerable difficulty as we wish to respect learning disabled people and their parents equally within our work. We feel we must not only listen, and afford acceptance to, the understandings of childhood status expressed by parents, but also entail recognition of legal, political, personal and social meanings ascribed to adulthood which frame persons over the age of 18 as not children. We need to avoid a fixed, unilinear view of 'the child' in order not to become ethnocentric and devaluing of different familial structures. But there are occasions, too, when a flexible, multilinear description of childhood would be unworkable.

Whose rights?

These matters bring us round to complicated entitlement issues which are bewildering when we are thinking about disabled children's rights. In studies involving children, what exactly does the notion of 'rights' and the concept of 'entitlement' mean in relation to the research act? Assumptions about children's rights are often treated uncritically as if there is universal consensus about what is acceptable and what is unacceptable, whereas each individual disability researcher will actually have personal, intuitive and culture bound preferences about the rights of children in disability projects. There is, however, no clearly established cornerstone against which to measure the validity or appropriateness of one's values and beliefs.

When we attempt to clarify what we mean by a 'rights view of a child' we are compelled to acknowledge the highly idiosyncratic resources which we each personally draw upon in the process – as daughters ourselves, as mothers, as sisters, as disabled or non-disabled women – and so on. Our own expectations of children's rights include the right to be heard, and moreover the right to be listened to. We have already made public our commitment to the United Nations Convention on the Rights of the Child (UNICEF 1995), which views a child's right to be listened to as an intrinsic part of the right to justice for each individual child and for children as a group within society (Moore *et al.* 1996). A child's right to be consulted is important to us, as is the child's right to have personal views taken seriously. These latter rights are especially pertinent in relation to situations or events which directly affect disabled children yet are often disguised, such as to do with explanations of physical limitations or plans for hospitalization or surgery (Todd and Shearn 1997). All children should have the right to a full and decent life, although what this means precisely we cannot say as we can comment only within the boundaries of our own knowledge and experience. The right to dignity, self-reliance, self-determination, respect, tolerance, and to participation and inclusion in the life of one's own community, are others which we ourselves prioritize. We sense that researchers should always be moving towards re-evaluation and new possibilities when specifying what their personal bill of children's rights would look like, and are conscious that a well-informed statement of those rights has to be continually evolving.

Historically, within the UK there is incessant struggle to clarify rights for children (Leach 1994; Franklin 1995). There are areas of gross ambiguity, for example, where parental choice is elevated over and above children's rights (Newell 1995). Also, the 1995 Disability Discrimination Act has proved instrumental in the undermining of disabled children's rights, failing to put into place rights for disabled children not to be discriminated against in terms of educational provision with justification being provided through pressure on resources (Scope 1997). There are also areas which lack clarity in the law, such as in the 1989 Children Act where a child's right to choose to be registered as disabled for example, or to receive an assessment, depends on whether the child is judged to be 'of sufficient understanding' (Smith 1994: 16). What exactly is meant by this is unclear and also based on a deficit view, rather than a rights based view, of the child. Such half-hearted recognition of children's rights is pervasive and this impinges on any research involving children. As a society, we may pay lip-service to a rhetoric of children's rights, but without prioritizing their own viewpoints and concerns we have little hope of recognizing their rights.

In our research, the dynamics of children's rights issues have become particularly explicit in relation to securing their access to a research project. We have found that the imbalance of power which exists between children and adults usually functions to determine a child's access to, or alienation from, the research process. This is a complex area for discussion.

In our study of children's reflections on family life, we were embroiled in the issues of how family predilections might restrict or impose upon the rights of a child as soon as we started setting up interviews (Beazley and Moore

1996). We found that even when attempts are made to invite children to participate in projects in their own right, the issue of consent is opaque. In this study, our initial approach was to parents and hence any expression of interest in the project and subsequently any decision to participate, or desist, was not explicitly the child's. Rather, children's consent was a product of the attitudes their parents held towards our work. If parents had not been willing to support what we were doing, we could not legitimately have tried to involve their children. Clearly a child's right to be heard is easily diluted. As parents, commenting from a different viewpoint, we know and understand that parents value their right to monitor the access researchers have to their children.

Attempts to obtain direct agreement from children prior to commencement of the interviews, despite good intentions to try and provide them with real choice, simply materialized as formalities in our study because permissions had already been given by a parent. This meant a child might have agreed to take part to please or appease a parent. Conversely, a child could have refused to participate in order to exert independence from a parent and not through lack of interest in project. The researcher can only surmise. For example, one of the teenage children with Deaf parents due to meet for a research interview was not there at the appointed time. His sister talked much about her concerns over her brother's rebellion against their parents especially as he seemed to be using the difference in communication modes to register his independence:

> Well, he's not good at signing. He gets impatient and mum can't understand what he's saying because he doesn't talk with his mouth . . . then she gets angry because he's getting impatient because she doesn't know what he's said.
>
> I think he likes to take advantage of my mum and dad because of them being deaf.

Tensions such as these are common in many families, including non-disabled families, and may muddy the likely reasons for involvement or otherwise in research. Tom Shakespeare (1997) also draws attention to the difficulties created when parents take on the role of speaking for their child. We have already noted this as part of a larger problem of disempowerment if the views of children and their parents clash, or if parents believe that their offspring are inarticulate or otherwise unable to contribute to the research process.

It seems a vexed question to put parents' and children's rights in juxtaposition and ask which should have precedent. Parental responsibility is defined in the 1989 Children Act as 'all rights, responsibilities and authority which by law a parent of a child has in relation to the child and her/his property' (Smith 1994: 5). However, the Act also states that courts should respond to the Paramountcy Principle, that is, 'if the interests of the child conflict with those of parents/others, the child's are of overriding importance'(Smith 1994: 2). How these conflicting interests are to be weighed up remains uncertain.

The community frequently questions the boundaries between such rights and responsibilities for children and parents and, particularly with regard to disabled children, some feel that the balance remains too far with the parents (Newell 1995). The debate echoes many themes of relevance to disability researchers working with children. An interesting example of where a wider community has commented on this balance of rights has arisen with regard to the use of cochlear implants (devices implanted within the ear to provide electrical stimulation of the acoustic nerve) with hearing impaired children:

> Who 'owns' the child? 'Ownership' is not a good word – 'responsibility' may be a better word, except that 'belonging' goes with 'ownership'. When children are old enough to take responsibility for decisions about themselves the situation becomes easier. . . . Parents feel the child belongs to them, they have a right and duty to make the best possible decisions for their child, for themselves, and for the whole family unit. Many, but not all, d/Deaf people feel that the children, by their deafness, are from birth part of the Deaf community and the community has duties and privileges in relation to the children.
>
> (Woodford 1995: 24)

Further, 'it cannot be said that parents are allowed to make an informed choice because so much of what they know about deafness [and] d/Deaf people . . . is based upon negative stereotypes' (Daniels 1995: 20).

Exactly who is in a position to make an informed choice is a question that has consistently plagued our disability research with children. We saw this in Chapter 2, where permission to observe children was controlled by school managers and teachers, while parents had only limited decision-making power over their child's involvement. The question of who had the right to give or withhold consent for children to participate in the project was laid wide open when one teacher wished pupils she regarded as 'hers' – because they were in her class – to be withdrawn from the project, even though their parents were happy for them to take part. The reverberations of power relations on children's access to research are plainly phenomenal.

Children's real right to choose is unclear, not only with regard to consent to become involved in a research project, but also in other aspects of the process. We can highlight many problem areas. How meaningful is it, for example, to give children control over the research agenda or methodology? What, for example, would a child make of the difference between being interviewed or observed? We have consistently found that when research participants of any age are asked for comments or ideas about methodology they are accepting of the researcher's choices and feel ill equipped for dictating a preference. This may be a result of inadequacies in personal and social education, especially where disabled children have soaked up feelings of low self-esteem through segregated schooling (Swain 1993). This issue, of the efficacy and value of collaboration with participants over research design, should not be oversimplified. Does the rhetoric of involving disabled people in all aspects of methodological decision-making extend to disabled children? If not, why not, and what are the implications?

There are further questions to ask when underway with interviewing, observing, experimental procedures or whatever the chosen methodology turns out to be. How can researchers ensure that parents remain as near as the child wants them, but are not intrusive? Is there any sense in worrying about these questions if, for example, child participants are babies or toddlers? Where does one draw the line? Again, children's rights are at the heart of this issue. Some concerns contradict others we have mentioned, such as the child's right to be with a parent during the course of investigative proceedings, and to have the parent speak for a child who feels shy or overwhelmed. All of these issues are extremely difficult to unravel. Another question, of considerable gravity, concerns whether researchers should ever bypass parents in order to access the perspectives of their children. Are there any circumstances in which researchers might legitimately circumvent parents to give voice to a child? What about in situations of known, or suspected abuse?

Returning to the observation study reported in Chapter 2 helps to bring some of the above-mentioned controversies into prominence. The Deaf father of a 3-year-old child being studied decided to accompany her during scheduled observation sessions. His reasons for this were twofold. First, as the child was the only BSL user in a largely non-signing environment, her father was worried that on an ordinary school day, the observer would be sure to record a great many failed communication attempts involving his daughter, which could be used to make a case for moving her to a segregated school. To counteract this, he wanted to be with her as facilitator of her interactions when observations were taking place, so that the researcher would record many instances of easy and effective communication. Second, he wanted to be around in order to satisfy himself that neither the observer nor the observation process intruded upon his child's school day. Researchers have choices in situations like this, between dismay at potential distortion of the picture of children's experiences, or being heartened by the resistance being shown towards unacceptable levels of interference by non-disabled researchers into disabled people's lives. But the situation is very much further complicated by the need to consider the child's own perspective in all of this. How would the issues be different if the child was not 3, attending preschool nursery, but 13, attending secondary school? What if a child did not want the parent around? Whose rights would the researcher be seeking to prioritize in this scenario? How could the rights of both the child and the parent be protected? Where do the commitments of researchers lie?

There are countless other issues to ponder. Who owns raw data such as video or audio tapes and transcripts? What are the functions of transcript ownership to a child who may not be literate, or of possession of audio recordings for a hearing impaired child? Do researchers, or parents, own raw data? Does a parent (any parent in particular?) have a right to read a child's transcript or to view tapes of the child's behaviour in school? Children might, for example, understand their antics in the playground to occupy a private space to which their parents do not have access. What happens if researchers acquire video-taped evidence of behaviour that might incriminate a child, yet which is incidental to the researchers' intended and stated purposes? One of

us met with this problem when filming children for evidence of their prag-
matic communication skills and recorded, in the process, long episodes of vio-
lent and aggressive behaviour which could have been used to occasion an
exclusion order. In this example, where do a child's rights begin and end? Can
6-year-old children who experience difficulty with communication grasp any
meaningful understanding of why they are being filmed for research into language development, let alone comprehend the potential misuses and abuses
of ensuing data? What are the researchers' responsibilities, and how do these
compare with obligations, in such situations?

These quandaries lead us back to the question of precisely whose permissions are required when disability research touches upon children's lives? We
have come across contentious and grey areas here, notably when setting up
interviews with children whose parents were separated. Usually we have settled for permission from the parent with custody of the child, but sometimes
parents have joint custody and do not share the same view of their child's
involvement in the research. On one occasion, where only one parent had
given permission for a child to participate because the other was estranged,
debates about ownership of the child's transcript took on the significance of
nightmares when the consenting parent realized its potency as evidence to
present against the former partner to the Child Support Agency. We have
made very little headway in finding any resolution for these dilemmas, and
repeatedly find ourselves dealing with each case according to its particular circumstances. Such questions remain important, however; researchers must
continually interrogate their own practice if children's rights in research are
to be even superficially endowed.

Thinking points

How can disabled children be offered equal access to equal opportunities in a research project? How can they give or refuse their consent? What issues need to be addressed? What progress can you make
towards enhancing children's rights within disability research by starting to identify any professional biases or personal assumptions about
possibilities for researching with children? How can you ensure that
you retain a sufficiently broad and open view of disabled children's
potential contributions to research? How can disabled children help
you to make your disability research practice more enabling?

Confidentiality

Alongside considerations to do with consent are equally cloudy questions
about confidentiality. Though researchers recognize the ethical and moral
implications of confidentiality, very often, the 'right to know', the 'need to
know' and the 'want to know' become confused and fudged on a day to day

basis (Maelzer 1995). Privacy and personal control are often glossed over, denied or forgotten by researchers and sometimes paid too little attention by those in positions of power over a child, including friends, relatives and professionals.

The complexities of 'confidential' versus 'anonymous', and 'private' versus 'secret' contributions, create anxiety for researchers working with children. To avoid some of the obvious pitfalls we explain to child participants that we will give them a pretend name in anything we write, or if we speak about them. We also emphasize that 'you can tell anyone you like about what we say. I will keep what you say private, but you can choose to tell other people if you want'. These strategies do not, of course, avoid potential conflict between a child and a parent if anyone can be recognized in an oral, signed or written account.

Sometimes we have felt that it would be too much of a breach of trust to compromise a child's anonymity if there would be problems caused by parents and other family members recognizing the child. One strategy is to relate experiences in a very general way, but this has to be done in the full knowledge that there will be gaps when experiences cannot be related to context. We exclude data, as a matter of course, if a child indicates that it is not for public airing, though this is never easy to determine, and results in partial accounts becoming even more partial. In addition, excluded material may be that which researchers would themselves most wish to afford public recognition, and is often material that reveals oppression in one guise or another. What action should researchers take if they do not *believe* that a child saying 'you won't tell anyone that will you?' actually means this to happen? We can ensure anonymity from the general readership, in terms of what the children say and how we report it. However, we cannot ensure confidentiality if we give too much personal detail for any child, and the in-depth nature of the qualitative accounts we favour makes identity very transparent. We remain conscious that all of these issues, while addressed to the best of our capability, are not fully resolved and require further debate and consideration by researchers as they work with children.

The final power relationship we wish to explore is that between researcher and child.

Researcher positions

There are problems about the relationship of the researcher with disabled children, and as Griffin (1995) suggests, it is difficult to conduct any form of investigative process without a degree of power differential between researcher and researched. Where children are involved, the problem is immense. Typically, in newly forged relationships, children often try to please and so defer to adults. This is something we have tried to reduce to a minimum during our research conversations but we remain aware that it exists and is yet another influence on the degree to which children's views can be reflected. Sometimes children may have told us what they think we wanted to know; there have also been times when we suspect that they have worked out what they think we want to get at and decided that we are not going to hear it. In one interview, in which we were genuinely interested in the child's experience of spilt-family life, we felt sure that the child taking part suspected us of prevaricating and really wanting to talk about disability, which was the usual focus of interest when professionals had anything to do with her. This child produced rich and thoughtful answers to everything we asked her about, and her transcript reveals that she thought equally hard about what she left out, as about what she put in. This reminds us of the necessity never to underestimate children's abilities and possibilities.

Adults occupying positions of power over children's participation in research may also try to please and defer to researchers. During our in-schools research, for example, staff have often asked our opinions about children and events. Some of these questions impact directly on the nature of data available. Again, from the study of inclusion described in Chapter 2, a teacher might ask 'shall I get the musical instruments out so you can see a d/Deaf and a hearing child playing together?' Such concessions to what is imagined to be the researcher's interests are hazardous because they disempower key players in the research situation (in this case teachers), they interfere with children's experiences (in this case for reasons of politeness rather than pedagogy) and they reduce the researchers' confidence that they are researching what they set out to research. Possibly such tensions could be avoided if researchers disguise their presence, but we feel strongly that the attendant ethical problems that would go with not revealing one's role far outweigh any advantages of covert investigation with children.

Once we have managed to explain our research plans to children, how do disability researchers then engage those children with research methodologies? Taking the case of interviews, as adults who have become reasonably skilled in the art of communication, it could be easy to lose sight of the linguistic, cognitive and interpersonal demands facing children in conversation. These demands are compounded by impairment for many children who do not find it easy to be understood when they interact with researchers who are strangers and may not be practised in their preferred mode of conversation. We have had to think carefully about setting 'communication ground-rules' when conducting group meetings with disabled children, to ensure that every child has equal access to the discussion, and to keep ourselves mindful that special receptive strategies and expressive skills are required of us. We find it helpful to have a flexible approach to communication with children. Mostly an informal, friendly everyday conversational style seems to work best, and we often play or draw with children in order to minimize the formality of the research situation.

When communicating via interpreters, the issues of equality, self-determination and respect merit special consideration in relation to a child's input to a discussion. When parents, friends or siblings, for instance, take on the interpreter role, how does this affect what a child can say? Their accounts will be compromised by their assessment of what they are comfortable with the interpreter knowing. Where a researcher combines interpreting with their researcher role, as has been the case in many of our studies where funding has been scarce, how does this compromise the child's rights? We know from experience that adopting this dual role detracts from the level of control a Deaf child (and the same is true for Deaf adults) can exert over the proceedings, and so they are disadvantaged in terms of choices and independence. It has been argued, and we agree, that professionals should not permit their roles to be confused in this way, and that Deaf people must be enabled to communicate without hindrance in their own language (Moorhead 1991), but as researchers who are constantly researching on a shoe-string budget, we have had to face the fact that the ideal world of disability research is not the same as the real one in which we operate. We offer this point not as an excuse, but to emphasize that researchers are subject to forms of oppression too, and none of us can operate from outside of our oppressive world. We share with other writers the conviction that for disabled children where communication barriers may exist, researchers must make continued efforts to guarantee both their inclusion in research, and representation of their views, as a matter of utmost urgency (Bench 1992; Mason 1995).

This debate about the insidious workings of power relations within research highlights the problems with determining children's 'best interests' which may be further accented where children for reasons of age or impairment, are less able to make their own opinions clear. Finally, the whole issue of funding is one that is relevant to all projects but we have chosen to raise questions of economics here because some of the general issues relating to financing of disability projects are more conspicuous in relation to studies involving children.

Economics and disabled children's research

It is in the context of economics and disabled children's research that we most readily encounter the problem mentioned at the start of this chapter whereby disability researchers working with children can produce dependency. The funding of studies of disabled children is often a source of pathologization. Funding agencies wield considerable power over the nature of research activity and may – intentionally or unintentionally – direct researchers to participate in pathologization of the lives of children with impairments, particularly if funds originate through benevolent agencies, which are not run by disabled people.

Researchers are obliged to wrestle with the contradictions between raising funds for a project and avoiding sources of funding which appeal to, and perpetuate, oppressive images of disabled children. Decisions about which funding applications to make involve a great deal of soul searching and we do need to acknowledge the self-interest of the researchers in these matters. We have on one occasion explicitly been confronted with some of these difficulties in our own pursuit of research moneys, and we found ourselves about to reconceptualize a proposal on the advice of external reviewers, in ways which we realized would mean carrying out research which fitted much more with ways in which funding bodies would regulate disabled children's lives, than with ways in which disabled people might chose to regulate – and produce knowledge about – their own lives.

The fate of the original proposal, which was submitted for an exploration of support networks for d/Deaf children, their families and professionals, is illustrative. The main concern expressed by reviewers was 'is [the project] value for money?' We know that this is a sensible consideration in the context of allocating limited resources for research. But when the query was unpicked it became clear that, in the reviewer's opinion, 'good use of broad written surveys' would provide a 'far more economical way' (and therefore more acceptable to the funding body) of accessing the views of d/Deaf children than research methods which sought to maximize empowerment opportunities for participants. Research strategies likely to produce minimal challenge to social practices ('broad written survey' techniques for accessing the views of d/Deaf children unquestionably came into this category) were deemed more likely to attract research funding. When we realized that getting the funding from this source would oblige us to issue standardized questionnaires to children who may well be struggling with written forms of communication, we acknowledged that it would be pointless to resubmit the proposal after all.

We have repeatedly found that research methods which are explicitly partisan, in the sense of giving disabled people and their nominated representatives control over both research production and outcomes, are not readily supported by the major research councils. Voluntary agencies and charities prove more likely sources of funding for disability research which involves children, but research findings produced through their offices are less visible to policy-makers and the powers that be. Some charitable organizations are so bound up with the creation of dependency that it is impossible to reconcile empowerment with their view of relevant disability research, and we have ourselves withdrawn from receipt of funding on offer from Children In Need for this reason. There has been a price to pay for turning down funding within the university sector, where external research income is used as an indicator of esteem (Higher Education Funding Council 1996), but we have counted this against the cost of demonstrating commitment to the articulations of disabled people on these matters. There is, nevertheless, some urgency for disability researchers to evolve concrete strategies to avoid tying up research support with either the charity business – which can bring associated pitiable and pathetic imagery (Barnes 1992; Burman 1996) – or with conventional sources of funding and associated emphasis on the production of non-partisan data of little practical or policy relevance to disabled people.

Questions of economics in the construction of research concerning disabled children do potentially give rise to oppression. The dilemma that researchers currently face often amounts to a choice between carrying out bland, yet relatively powerful research with research council funding which provides financial back-up for correspondingly prosaic dissemination, or to carry out more partial projects either unfunded, or funded by charities, which are meaningful to service users yet have more tenuous capacity for bringing about change. Research relating to disabled children's lives frequently does attract the support of charitable organizations, but there is a paradox here because when resourced through these assets investigations of disabled children's lives risk being smothered by assumptions about dependency and, in addition, are usually impairment linked.

That there is disillusion with existing forms of funding for critical disability research generally, and projects involving disabled children specifically, is a message which we have often heard repeated. It can be argued that economic practices surrounding research comprise a powerful source of oppression and so, what we have learned, is that researchers must, of necessity, keep asking questions about sources of funding and trying to challenge oppressive economic acts.

Conclusions

This chapter has primarily been about disability research which involves children and the risks of pathologization and oppression of children both within society and in research. We believe that researchers need to be willing to challenge stereotypical assumptions often made about how disabled children can (or cannot) contribute to the research process and we hope this chapter will widen and stimulate discussion of children's possibilities. It is essential that researchers carrying out studies of disabled children and their childhoods are aware of the complexities involved, and also recognize that there are no easy answers. The aspiration to emancipatory disability research involving children demands much rethinking of relations between researchers and those being researched, and children's rights issues exacerbate many of the difficulties described elsewhere in this book. In the concluding chapter we point to the importance of continuing to ask critical questions as part of the process of continually shaking up one's assumptions and representations of disabled people's lives.

Thinking points

List some of the rights you consider as essential for disabled children involved in a research project. Why have you listed these? How does your personal, professional and political experience influence the list? Critically review some recent research papers in the area of disability and childhood in order to clarify your thoughts on what a bill of children's rights in research should preserve. What mechanisms can be put in place to ensure that the rights you prioritize are safeguarded within your own investigations? Consider the reasons why issues concerning children's rights in the research process are important for understanding any person's rights entitlement in disability research.

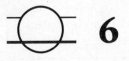 **6**

Developing new pathways for disability researchers

Introduction

In this concluding chapter we comment on the emergent themes from the book and attempt to reiterate and clarify our general concerns about advancing an agenda for critical disability research. Many of the threads that run through the chapters are drawn together to provide an overview of the key issues that concern disability researchers and the implications of these for research practice. Some of the most important lessons revealed by our experiences of research are highlighted. The implications of concerns raised by each chapter will be reviewed. As the descriptive detail of our research undertakings will necessarily be missing here, readers may wish to return to the accounts to supplement this review. Next, suggestions are made about how we might respond to the variety of challenges which arise for disability researchers. This leads on to discussion of issues involved in creating alliances between disabled and non-disabled people in research since we believe this shapes the future research process and will provide for the emergence of relevant research productions through which disabled people's experiences are more and more meaningfully evaluated.

We hope it is evident that our main purpose in writing this book has not been to prescribe a clear, consolidated way to conduct disability research nor to dictate to other researchers a definitive means of approaching their projects. What we have intended is to provide reflective accounts of our experiences, good and ill, as researchers grappling with the enormity of trying to understand the human rights issues involved in projects focusing on disability. We have stated our belief several times, that being critical about ourselves in terms of values, assumptions, practices and personal and professional development is an essential aspect of an emancipatory approach to disability research. We have tried to be open and honest and engage with appropriate ethical frameworks, but must admit to finding the high degree of self-exposure tremendously

taxing. Presumably, many readers will recognize themselves in similarly problematic situations, and will realize that by taking this opportunity to be reflexive in a public domain, and hence in association with others, we are trying to
prompt a move beyond academic discussion, towards practical ways forward.
As we reach this juncture, we want now to review the utility of the accounts
provided and to consider ideas about ways forward.

What this book has been about

The successes and failures of a variety of research projects have been chron-
icled in order that the reader might gain insight into the complexities of conducting research in the shadow of the politics and power games which are
by-products of the professional and vocational structures surrounding disabled people. Despite the different settings and activities under consideration,
it is notable that they raise similar issues about disability research practice.
They all point to the dangers of inadequate inclusion of the people whose
quality of life an investigation is meant to elucidate or improve. It is evident
that researchers have to weigh up many things in the process of setting up
projects; asking not only themselves, but also those who are the focus of their
inquiries what the research is for, who is to benefit from it, what tangible outcomes the investigation will produce and how it is intended to be used. Well
thought out plans for dissemination turn out to be crucial if the research is to
make an impact and if disabled people who collaborate with researchers can
be assured that disabling barriers which they help to identify are to be dis-
mantled. Important opportunities exist for researchers to assist in the promotion of self-determination of those with whom the research is concerned,
but only if a relentlessly critical approach to inquiry is adopted. We try to sum-
marize some of the lessons we have learned.

Alliances against 'hijack'

Through reflection on traditional research practice, characterized by the conventional commitments by which researchers are expected to abide, we discovered just how easily a piece of research can be 'hijacked', misused and
abused. It was surprising to an uninitiated non-disabled postgraduate research
student to discover just how virulently non-disabled professionals might
oppose the emancipation of disabled people and how those with sufficient
power can relentlessly manipulate the research process, the researcher and
the researched, to further their own oppressive personal and political interests. Abuses ranged from reification of the concept of objectivity as a strategy
for excluding disabled people from engagement with research, to denial of the
rights of disabled children to use their own language in the research setting.
All of the projects we have presented met with some opposition from non-
disabled service providers who wished to ignore the priorities of disabled

people and use the projects for their own purposes and gain. It became clear that researchers must work together with disabled people in order to begin to get around such obstacles in the pursuit of research and empowerment.

An important dimension of the reflective commentaries was the sense of powerlessness that non-disabled researchers have, when they misguidedly (though sometimes for reasons outside of their control) find themselves doing research which is intended to advance the interests of disabled people, yet takes place without disabled people or members of their representative agencies as allies. Only more recently, by working as co-researchers with disabled people, have those of us who are the non-disabled writers begun to rediscover the positive side of research activity which leads to implementation of changes which disabled people want (Beazley *et al.* 1997; Skelton *et al.* 1997; Maelzer *et al.* 1998; Moore, Patient and Skelton 1998). The issue of the research agenda being overpowered and rendered oppressive of disabled people by non-disabled people in positions of control is clearly addressed in Chapters 2, 3 and 4.

Gaining support through a collaborative approach to inquiry, in which investigations are conducted alongside service users and service providers in tandem, is one way of developing a more emancipatory research approach. This was the strategy reported in Chapter 3. However, when researchers are positioned as go-betweens, trying to harmonize the interests of service users and service providers separately, rather than being able to bring the two groups together, this can cause confusion and conflict. Thus we have reflected on the need for researchers to challenge 'expert' knowledge of professionals and to tighten up our acknowledgement and understanding of the damage non-disabled people can do to disabled people's lives through research. When researchers have divided loyalties between service providers and users they meet with many drawbacks. We saw that the power balance in service-related research is almost always weighted on the side of the service providers who have their own agendas and vested interests in the results. Thus, in Chapter 3, we saw research findings skewed by non-disabled professionals and the rights of the disabled school leavers much diminished. Another clear example of this could be seen in Chapter 4, when a family support worker seemed set on sabotaging the promotion of service improvements which parents of disabled children wished to set in motion through their participation in research interviews. We have attempted to break some of the silence surrounding the personal and political complications which almost always seem to encroach on disability research projects.

Commitment to solidarity

The theme of commitment has recurred throughout the book and has been chosen to describe our changing understandings of approaches to disability research. Not only is a researcher's commitment to the agendas of disabled people essential, but also it must be established from the earliest conception of every project. We found that when commitment to a partisan approach is clarified during the course of a project, this is usually too late; non-disabled people may have been quick to monopolize crucial aspects of the design and planning of the research with the consequence that considerable creativity and post-project consultancy with disabled people and their representative allies is needed to rectify the situation and to protect against marginalization of disabled people's own priorities. While imaginative thinking can guard against further alienation where input from disabled people has been minimal during the course of a project, compensatory strategies are not seen as part of a truly emancipatory approach. It is inevitable that even well-intentioned projects cannot always be operationalized in ways which disability researchers know to be ideal, but this is not to say that oppressive practices within research can sometimes be tolerated. Researchers and disabled people need to offer one another support, characterized by Hurst (1995) as 'the support of solidarity', if empowerment of disabled people through research is not to be denied.

It is interesting to note that the processes that underlie critical disability research were similar across the focal projects. We gather that it is possible to mould and embellish research activity to suit the agenda of disabled people, even in the face of resistance, if researchers have carved out some opportunities for disabled people to play an influential role. Ideally, however, each project needs to be sufficiently well conceptualized to position disabled people centrally as co-researchers from the outset. In the project involving d/Deaf school leavers, d/Deaf consultants and young disabled people showed their own commitment to research outcomes by suggesting ways of promoting the findings with a view to bringing about change in their own lives. Although some of the service providers who collaborated on various projects did not seem convinced or impressed by the findings, their involvement did clarify the need to ensure that disability research is fully committed to disabled people *first*.

It was clear from the very real conflicts of interest that we have been caught up in, that employment of the medical model of disability in research invariably functions to substantiate the credibility of services and service providers. This has secured our commitment to developing research practice based on a social model of disability. We have laid open the futility of our attempts to side with disabled people from within an organization preoccupied with promoting its own self-interests through research based on the medical model of disability. Coming through the difficulties of researching with people who are unwilling to relinquish the medical model has helped us to fashion a sense of ourselves as autonomous disability researchers, and has underlined many paradoxes and survival strategies that researchers need to confront as part of their regular activity.

Practical resistance

We have frequently had to appeal to disabled people for assistance in resisting complicated abuses of power within a research situation. There have been a few episodes when we have had to relinquish the safety of the prospect of acquiring funding for our research in order to retain independence and control. Striking out without financial back-up has precipitated us into the business of practical resistance of oppression and has sometimes instituted more of a struggle than we had anticipated, such as when two of us resigned, rather than help to recycle disempowerment through research. However, once researchers are thrust into the midst of the battle to resist disempowerment, it is possible to uncover new networks which will better facilitate the proper role of disabled people in research about their lives.

Perhaps one of the most difficult messages of this book concerns the importance of evolving direct action against tendencies towards oppression in disability research. In several of the projects described, we reached the point where organizational and attitudinal barriers, and also those long developing institutional barriers which prevent disabled people from expressing views and making decisions were fully recognized, but we were then at a loss to know how to deal with such a stultifying situation.

All of this points to the need for researchers to consider ways of applying theoretical understandings of the importance of change to the situations they are working in. This may help to preserve the importance of small advances and strategies for moving a static atmosphere forward. Part of this involves disability researchers in learning how to empower themselves as an essential part of the process of facilitating the empowerment of others. It is easy to become impeded by some of the disillusionment that comes with facing up to what really goes on in the name of research which impacts on disabled people's lives. Researchers often find themselves personally disempowered during the course of a project, and it is important to take stock of the implications of this for both the research context in which they are operating, and for the disabled people with whose lives the project is connected.

One of the most practical aspects of our reflections on research is recognition that the interpersonal dynamics in working research groups are of utmost importance. This book might appropriately be subtitled '*Research and Biscuits*' as testimony to the emphasis that we place on trying to set up positive working relations. Differing perspectives can be exciting and challenging, bringing new ways of channelling ideas, but divergent goals, philosophies and means of responding to conflicting pressures can be disastrous, slowing the research process down or even bringing it to a complete standstill. Inclusion of disabled people and other stakeholders in all discussions about the research seems to be a fundamentally important step towards keeping a research group focused. Other mechanisms, such as the shared formulation of the rights of those participating in the research process, also need to be identified and agreed in order to deal with potential difficulties in such contexts. It is worth mentioning that working together in a team with disabled and non-disabled researchers brings its own pressures and we shall focus on these later on in this discussion.

Before diverging from discussion of practical resistance of disempowerment in disability research it is worth reminding ourselves that in several chapters we have disclosed uncertainties about where the commitments of disability researchers working with children should lie. We have pondered the un-certain place of children's rights in general in society, and the effects this has for researchers, through looking at manifestations of complicated rights issues in some of our own work. There is a need to deconstruct – and to reconstruct – many assumptions about children and their childhoods and about the posi-tion of children in disability research. We cannot claim to provide any unan-imous resolutions to the special problems posed by involvement of children in disability research projects, but wanted to portray our concerns and per-haps prompt further debate.

Ways forward: defining and declaring rights

We are constantly trying to find better ways to work, which means further focus on identifying, bringing to the fore and trying to embody within pro-jects, the rights that we feel disabled people should have within research. We cannot profess to hold the key to the definitive way of ensuring that research is always conducted in an equal and non-oppressive way for disabled people. Attitudes pervading society at large (Barnes 1990; Morris 1991; Zarb 1995; Campbell and Oliver 1996; Oliver 1996) are changing only slowly and train-ing for professionals (including research training) remains largely based upon the medical model with its allegiance to positivist modes of inquiry. However, at this stage in our ever-evolving approach, we do have some thoughts about the ways we see for moving ourselves forward.

For research to begin to take account of the rights that disabled people have within a project which is focused upon them, the whole process from proposal to dissemination and implementation needs to respond to those rights as the researchers see them. Some short but overt statement of the rights which the researchers hold dear could be defined at the start of each project, this then acting as a clear message to others about the researchers' commitments. Immediately this seems to be no easy route, with disagreements emerging even before the project has begun. This declaring of one's personal bill of rights seems to us essential, but is not intended to impinge upon the rights that other people assume for themselves.

It seems imperative that researchers be honest from the start about their own values because these shape the whole research process – agenda setting, methodology, dissemination, empowerment prospects and so on. Hence, in our view, there is considerable obligation to declare one's own starting points. This can be harrowing if such declaration alienates the researchers from cer-tain potential, and powerful, participants, such as key service providers, per-haps even to the extent that the opportunity to pursue the research might be lost altogether. But we feel that if all research participants can be openly and honestly made aware of assumptions which researchers bring with them, then the pitfalls of becoming embroiled in a situation which might compromise the rights of disabled people can be reduced, and (through bitter experience) we have learned that this is imperative. In addition, where stakeholders do challenge researchers' own starting points, this can usefully encourage debate, stimulate the gathering of ammunition to defend an argument, or at best facilitate consideration of change. Often, too, personal disclosure is reciprocated thus providing the opportunity of knowing the commitments of others.

It has been established that any declaration of rights that researchers might produce can only be a product of their own formulation of current ideals in relation to a particular issue. It is important to recognize this fluctuating dimension to rights as this in itself can encourage others to take part in the debate rather than feeling threatened by any apparently strong ethical assertion being taken by researchers. Many things will sway the way in which disability researchers construe rights issues. Personal biography, ambition, regulation by funding bodies, professional monitoring and evaluation procedures and opportunities for developing self-awareness are just a few of the shaping factors – some of these more coercive than others. An explicit statement of rights could make disability researchers answerable in a more tangible way, leaving fewer bolt-holes for those operating – knowingly or not – in oppressive ways. When there are fewer places to hide, however, disability researchers can find themselves on uncertain territory, and to conclude we shall illustrate an instance of the effects this can have from our own experience, in order to show how the business of attending to the relations between disabled and non-disabled people within research is not tantamount to a guarantee of mutually acceptable joint participation.

Disabled and non-disabled alliances

Much of our reported research experience, together with the current literature on disability research, has pointed researchers and disabled people towards partnership approaches (Graves 1991; Zarb 1992; Lloyd *et al.* 1996; Sample 1996). We wish to suggest, however, that the notion of partnership may constitute the latest bandwagon for well-meaning, enthusiastic groups of disabled people and their non-disabled allies seeking to research together. We are in favour of a partnership approach that brings disabled and non-disabled people together, but are trying to place it within a stronger framework which has critical reflection on human rights at its foundation. Effective research relations between disabled and non-disabled researchers, must also, we feel, be constituted within this framework and will have to be worked at with great assiduity. But all will not simply be well just because disabled people and non-disabled people conduct research together; integrity and credibility have to be carefully established in relation to both academic rigour and political commitments.

Again, we find critical self-reflection revealing. Even in the last days of writing this book together, we are still learning that critical examination of rights within and beyond our own research team is a fundamental prerequisite for emancipatory research activity. Our final task as authors was to draw together ideas about how disabled people can agitate for proper representation and inclusion in research. The gist of what the one of us who is disabled had to say was as follows:

> Disabled people experiencing discrimination and exclusion can often find support for fighting against this within institutional rules and organizational and ethical guidelines for equal opportunities – often these just constitute words though – like we are writing in the book really – it's all very well saying these things about including disabled people and putting their views first, but it's what you do about it that really counts . . . in ordinary, informal research groups like ours, the disabled people have to continue to be up front and challenging all the time which is very hard. It's very tiring to be up front all of the time, it makes me feel vulnerable, there's always the risk of upsetting each other if every single thing which needs challenging is challenged. Sometimes you feel like giving up – but then you're giving in and having power taken away from you – but actually allowing power to be taken away – it all comes back to making challenging and cogent arguments about how you feel. Disabled people have to be assertive and ratty and bolshy, but more important perhaps than simply trying to be assertive, you have to make strong and cogent arguments about how you feel.

Reflexivity can lead to uncomfortable realizations, and Barton (1996) has pointed out that paving the way with good intentions provides no guarantee of successful routes forward. The above remarks highlight the persistence of inequities within our own research team and suggest that we have yet to overcome problems of isolation as a source of potential disempowerment within the working group. These reflections led on to recognition of difficulties within our approach to co-research and co-authorship, and now that we have this out in the open, we must work towards a mutually acceptable way of dismantling the identified barriers to equal participation.

Hence, commendable though the aim of forging alliances between disabled and non-disabled researchers may appear, we have to admit that it is a woolly and often time-consuming business, based on large amounts of nebulous factors such as 'good-will' and 'give and take'. Steps taken towards evolving participatory ways of working are consequently difficult to evaluate effectively. We have, with some trepidation, attempted to brave the specifics of this problem for these concluding remarks. Clearly, the one of us who is a disabled researcher at times feels excluded from our joint activities. But even though our alliance as a team of non-disabled and disabled researchers working together has come to be inspired by friendship and mutual respect first, and professionalism second, processes of continual critical reflection between ourselves are still not always easy.

A practical example which has emerged as an issue only in these last days relates to physical production of text. All too close to the deadline for the manuscript completion one of the non-disabled co-authors had to spend six distraught hours dealing with a virus on the word processor when what she really wanted to do in that time was to redraft a chapter. When this stressful episode was relayed to the disabled co-author, it materialized that six hours, each of them highly stressful due to the uncertainties of typing via personal assistants, was probably the time she needed to produce one page of text. While there had been a tacit acceptance of this, it now became possible to open up to each other about some aspects of joint writing. Again the gist of what emerged is revealing in terms of our own headway towards partici-patory ways of working:

> [over the phone] I'm so jealous to hear you typing all this . . . typing at a hundred words a minute. I suppose I'm comparing my speed to yours – there are real physical limitations to engagement with research processes for disabled people. Often these aren't seen, or aren't recognized – depending on other things that are going on at the time – other agendas which people might have – some people deliberately ignore our physical limitations and then use what they have chosen not to see as ammuni-tion for further marginalization of disabled people. It works both ways. The opposite is also true, like for us three writing this book. You are my co-researchers, and you do recognize my physical limitations and that makes me feel bad. I feel you are making excuses for what feels to me like my 'incompetence'. As a disabled person working with non-disabled people I tend to overcompensate in order to be 'as good as you' – I mean physically 'as good as' – spending loads more time than I have really got energy for, or pretending I haven't taken as long as I have taken – people do do that – it becomes a habit but we all do it.

It is essential that such issues are openly and regularly aired, but still it has taken us all several years of working together really to begin sharing these kinds of things properly. Ironically even talking about these issues in relation to ourselves was very hard, even though we were dealing with exactly the same points within the book. There is further irony in that the closer and more secure the relationships become between the three of us, the more will-ing we are to overcompensate for each other but this is irrespective of whether we are disabled or not, and the same reaction surfaces for a variety of reasons, such as to support each other through episodes of illness or ma-ternity leave.

The whole process of recognizing the strengths of individual members in any team, while also allowing for a flexible style which can accommodate the vagaries of differing demands and pressures on each at any one time, is a com-plex one. However, we now know that it cannot go unexplored in the hope that goodwill, mutual respect and shared commitment is sufficient. Positive and enabling relations between disabled and non-disabled people researching together are not based solely on friendly interpersonal dynamics. They stem from serious reflection on the social origins of disablement, they reside in commitment to mutual respect of each other's rights, and they are strength-ened through taking every opportunity to understand evolving research situ-ations in terms of theoretical accounts of the politics of disablement. If we had started from where we are now in our earlier research productions, then we might have produced rather more emancipatory disability research outputs than those which have been reviewed in this book.

Research that is truly aimed at empowerment and emancipation of disabled people would not only reduce the day to day experience of oppression experienced by individual disabled people, but also improve prospects for liberation and freedom from oppression for disabled people as a group and minimize the injustices that occur in any disabled person's life at any time. The pace of change in the nature of disability research production is currently rapid and increasing. We feel that there is an urgent need for wide-ranging discussions to develop a shared vision, not just of disability research processes, but of the sort of social and material changes that disabled people would prefer research to pursue and the policies that are needed to achieve this. Most importantly, we believe it is essential to place disabled people firmly at the forefront of such dialogue.

Final remarks

Throughout the book we have advocated a reflexive, self-analytical critical approach to disability research firmly grounded in human rights principles. It would be discouraging to imply that the route to this understanding in our disability research careers has been dismal and depressing. We have greatly valued our opportunities to progress a disability rights agenda based on disabled people's own priorities and, within this book, expanding and sharing a contribution to resourceful disability research practice. Likewise we have enjoyed the challenge of evolving critical directions in our research and finding ways of dismantling disabling barriers within and produced by our own activities. We have gained a great deal through trying to take up the quest for disability researchers to connect the personal to the political (Oliver 1996) but the personal and political realities of discovery have, at times, been painful. While our closing demand is for research to be enabling and empowering, this must not be seen as a soft option, an inferior or sheltered form of research activity. In terms of planning, procedures, analysis and outcomes, critical rights-based emancipatory disability research is, we feel, to be constituted with unequivocal rigour, and to be seen as an example of the variety of approaches to disability research that are necessary given the complexity of the human subject.

Finally, we feel that there is no room for complacency or for arrogance on the part of researchers. We are ever and always learners. We have so much to learn and to achieve that a position of humility and a desire to work with others in the demanding pursuit of critical, rights-based emancipatory is essential. We have found that disability research involves debate, listening and earning the respect of others, particularly in relation to the voices of disabled people. We hope that in the future disabled people participating in research alongside us will no longer need to ask, as they have done in the past, 'do you think what you are doing will make any change, make anything better?' We hope that as a team of disabled and non-disabled people working together, we shall be able to further evolve our research practice in ways which will enable disabled people to be instrumental in providing the answers themselves. It is now the readers' task to respond to these deliberations within their own disability research endeavours.

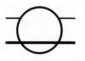

References

Abberley, P. (1987) The concept of oppression and the development of a social theory of disability, *Disability, Handicap and Society*, 2 (1): 5–21.

Abberley, P. (1992) Counting us out: a discussion of the OPCS disability surveys, *Disability, Handicap and Society*, 7 (2): 139–56.

Barnes, C. (1990) *Cabbage Syndrome: The Social Construction of Dependency*. London: Falmer Press.

Barnes, C. (1992) Qualitative research: valuable or irrelevant, *Disability, Handicap and Society*, 7 (2): 115–24.

Barnes, C. (1996) Disability and the myth of the independent researcher, *Disability and Society*, 11 (1): 107–10.

Barnes, C. (ed.) (1997) *Doing Disability Research*. Leeds: The Disability Press.

Barton, L. (ed.) (1988) *The Politics of Special Educational Need*. Lewes: Falmer Press.

Barton, L. (1996) *Disability and Society: Emerging Issues and Insights*. London: Longman.

Barton, L. and Clough, P. (1995) Conclusion: many urgent voices, in P. Clough and L. Barton (eds) *Making Difficulties: Research and the Construction of SEN*. London: Paul Chapman.

Beazley, S. and Moore, M. (1995) *Deaf Children, their Families and Professionals: Dismantling Barriers*. London: David Fulton.

Beazley, S. and Moore, M. (1996) Family lives of hearing children with Deaf parents, in M. Moore, J. Sixsmith and K. Knowles (eds) *Children's Reflections on Family Life*. London: Falmer Press.

Beazley, S., Moore, M. and Benzie, D. (1997a) Involving disabled people in research: A study of inclusion in environmental activities, in G. Mercer and C. Barnes (eds) *Doing Disability Research*. Leeds: The Disability Press.

Beazley, S., Moore, M., Benzie, D., Maelzer, J. and Patient, M. (1997b) *Researching Inclusion of Disabled People in Environmental Activities*. Report compiled on behalf of the Salford and Trafford Groundwork Trust by the Manchester Metropolitan University Disability Studies Team.

Beazley, S., Skelton, J. and Maelzer, J. (1998) *Learning Disabled People: Innovative Options for Living*. Lancaster: Venture Press.

Bench, J. (1992) *Communication Skills in Hearing-Impaired Children*. London: Whurr.

Billington, T. (1996) Pathologising children: psychology in education and acts of government, in E. Burman, G. Aitken, P. Alldred, R. Allwood, T. Billington, B. Goldberg, A. J. Gordo Lopez, C. Heenan, D. Marks and S. Warner, *Psychology Discourse Practice: From Regulation to Resistance*. London: Taylor and Francis.

Bradley, B. S. (1989) *Visions of Infancy*. Oxford: Polity/Blackwell.

Burman, E. (1994) *Deconstructing Developmental Psychology*. London: Routledge.

Burman, E. (1996) Constructing and deconstructing childhood: images of children and charity appeals, in J. Haworth (ed.) *Psychological Research: Innovative Methods and Strategies*. London: Routledge.

Burton, M. and Kagan, C. (1996) Rethinking empowerment: shared action against powerlessness, in I. Parker and R. Spears (eds) *Psychology and Society: Radical Theory and Practice*. London: Pluto Press.

Campbell, J. and Oliver, M. (1996) *Disability Politics: Understanding Our Past, Changing Our Future*. London: Routledge.

Clark, M. (1989) *Language through Living for Hearing-Impaired Children*. London: Hodder and Stoughton.

Clough, P. and Barton, L. (eds) (1995) *Making Difficulties: Research and the Construction of SEN*. London: Paul Chapman.

Connors, E. and Glenn, S. M. (1996) Methodological considerations in observing mother–infant interactions in natural settings, in J. Haworth (ed.) *Psychological Research: Innovative Methods and Strategies*. London: Routledge.

Corker, M. (1993) Integration and deaf people, in J. Swain, V. Finkelstein, S. French and M. Oliver (eds) *Disabling Barriers – Enabling Environments*. London: Sage in association with The Open University.

Daniels, S. (1995) Cochlear implants in the UK, *Cochlear Implant and Bilingualism*, Kimpton: LASER.

Edwards, A. and Talbot, R. (1994) *The Hard Pressed Researcher: A Research Handbook for the Caring Professions*. London: Longman.

Edwards, D. (1993) Practices and provisions for hearing-impaired children, in K. Mogford-Bevan and J. Sadler (eds) *Child Language Disability: Volume III*. Clevedon: Multilingual Matters.

Fish Report (1985) *Educational Opportunities for All? Report of the Committee Reviewing Provision to Meet Special Educational Needs*. London: Inner London Education Authority.

Foster, J. and Parker, I. (1995) *Carrying Out Investigations in Psychology: Methods and Statistics*. Leicester: British Psychological Society.

Franklin, B. (1995) *The Handbook of Children's Rights: Comparative Policy and Practice*. London: Routledge.

French, S. (1988) Dispelling the mystique surrounding research, *Therapy Weekly*, 14 April.

Graves, W. (1991) Participatory action research: a new paradigm for disability and rehabilitation research, ARCA Newsletter, September: 8–11.

Gregory, S., Bishop, J. and Sheldon, L. (1996) *Deaf Young People and their Families: Developing Understanding*. Cambridge: Cambridge University Press.

Griffin, C. (1995) Feminism, social psychology and qualitative research, *The Psychologist*, 8 (3): 119–21.

Hegarty, S. (1993) *Meeting Special Needs in Ordinary Schools*, 2nd edn. London: Cassell.

Higher Education Funding Council (1996) *Research Assessment Exercise: Criteria for Assessment*, Circular 3/95. Bristol: HEFC.

Hirst, M. and Baldwin, S. (1994) *Unequal Opportunities: Growing Up Disabled*. London: Social Policy Research Unit (HMSO).

Hogg, J. and Cavet, J. (1995) *Making Leisure Provision for People with Profound Learning and Multiple Disabilities*. London: Chapman Hall.

Homan, R. (1991) *The Ethics of Social Research*. London: Longman.

Hurst, R. (1995) Choice and empowerment – lessons from Europe, *Disability and Society*, 10 (4): 529–34.

In-Schools Project (1985) 'Field reports of the Avery Hill College In-Schools Research Team', unpublished paper, Avery Hill College, Special Educational Needs Section.

Jones, L. and Pullen, G. (1992) Cultural differences: deaf and hearing researchers working together, *Disability, Handicap and Society*, 7 (2): 189–96.

Kittel, R. (1991) Total commitment to total communication, in G. Taylor and J. Bishop (eds) *Being Deaf: The Experience of Deafness*. London: Pinter. (Original publication 1989.)

Ladd, P. (1988) The modern deaf community, in D. Miles (ed.) *British Sign Language*. London: BBC Publications Ltd.

Ladd, P. (1991) The erosion of social and self-identity, in G. Montgomery (ed.) *The Integration and Disintegration of the Deaf in Society*. Edinburgh: Scottish Workshop Publications. (Original publication 1981.)

Leach, P. (1994) *Children First*. Harmondsworth: Penguin.

Leadbetter, J. and Leadbetter, P. (1993) *Special Children: Meeting the Challenge in the Primary School*. London: Cassell.

Lloyd, M., Preston-Shoot, M., Temple, B. with Wuu, R. (1996) Whose project is it anyway? Sharing and shaping the research and development agenda, *Disability and Society*, 11 (3): 301–15.

Lynas, W. (1994) *Communication Options in the Education of Deaf Children*. London: Whurr.

Maelzer, J. (1991) 'June' in *Readings in Disability: Identity, Sexuality and Relationships*. Department of Health and Social Welfare. Milton Keynes: Open University.

Maelzer, J. (1995) 'Confidentiality', unpublished paper. Manchester Metropolitan University.

Maelzer, J., Moore, M. and Beazley, S. (1998) *Enabling Disabled Parents*. London: David Fulton.

Marks, D. (1996) Constructing a narrative: moral discourse and young people's experience of exclusion, in E. Burman, G. Aitken, P. Alldred, R. Allwood, T. Billington, B. Goldberg, A. J. Gordo Lopez, C. Heenan, D. Marks and S. Warner, *Psychology Discourse Practice: From Regulation to Resistance*. London: Taylor and Francis.

Mason, M. (1995) Inclusion: Empowering Disabled People. Conference Paper, Centre for Studies on Inclusive Education, the UN Convention on the Rights of the Child, UN Rules on Disabled People and UNESCO Statement on Inclusive Education, December, London.

McNiff, J. (1988) *Action Research: Principles and Practice*. London: Macmillan Education.

Miller, J. (1990) *Creating Spaces and Finding Voices*. New York: State University of New York Press.

Montgomery, G. (ed.) (1986) *Beyond Hobson's Choice: The appraisal of methods of teaching language to deaf children*. Edinburgh: Scottish Workshop Publications.

Moore, M. (1993) 'Opportunities for communication in integrated settings: young deaf children', unpublished PhD thesis. University of Greenwich.

Moore, M. and Beazley, S. (1995) 'The post-school reflections of young Deaf people', unpublished Manchester Polytechnic Research Report.

Moore, M., Patient, M. and Skelton, J. (1998) *Enabling Older Caregivers*. Lancaster: Venture Press.

Moore, M., Sixsmith, J. and Knowles, K. (eds) (1996) *Children's Reflections on Family Life*. London: Falmer Press.

Moorehead, D. (1991) Social work and interpreting, in S. Gregory and G. Hartley (eds) *Constructing Deafness*. London: Pinter.

Moorehead, D. (1997) Meanings of deafness. *Deaf Worlds: Deaf People, Community and Society*, 13 (1): 2–8.

Morris, J. (1991) *Pride Against Prejudice: Transforming Attitudes to Disability*. London: The Women's Press.

Morris, J. (1992a) Personal and political: a feminist perspective on researching physical disability, *Disability, Handicap and Society*, 7 (2): 157–66.

Morris, J. (ed.) (1992b) *Alone Together: Voices of Single Mothers*. London: The Women's Press.

National Deaf Children's Society (1993) Schools out: hopes and dreams on leaving school, *TALK*, 148, Summer: 18–21.

Newell, P. (1995) The Case for an End to Segregated Education. Conference Paper, Centre for Studies on Inclusive Education, the UN Convention on the Rights of the Child, UN Rules on Disabled People and UNESCO Statement on Inclusive Education, December, London.

Oliver, M. (1990) *The Politics of Disablement*. London: Macmillan.

Oliver, M. (1992) Changing the social relations of research production?, *Disability, Handicap and Society*, 7 (2): 101–14.

Oliver, M. (1993) Re-defining disability: a challenge to research, in J. Swain, V. Finkelstein, S. French and M. Oliver (eds) *Disabling Barriers: Enabling Environments*. London: Sage.

Oliver, M. (1996) *Understanding Disability: From Theory to Practice*. London: Macmillan.

Oliver, M. (1997) 'Emancipatory research: realistic goal or impossible dream', unpublished draft paper. University of Greenwich.

Rioux, M. and Bach, M. (eds) (1994) *Disability is Not Measles*. Ontario: Roeher Institute.

Riseborough, G. (1993) Recent policy, the numbers game and the schooling of the hearing-impaired: a study of one teacher's career, *European Journal of Special Needs Education*, 8 (2): 134–52.

Robinshaw, H. (1996) Acquisition of speech pre- and post-cochlear implantation: longitudinal studies of a congenitally deaf infant, *European Journal of Disorders of Communication*, 31 (2): 121–39.

Rose, C., Moore, M. and Howard, J. (1986) 'Personal and social education in a secondary school: a case study', unpublished Thames Polytechnic Research Report.

Sample, P. (1996) Beginnings: participatory action research and adults with developmental disabilities, *Disability and Society*, 11 (3): 317–32.

Scope (1997) *Schools Access Initiative Campaign*. London: Scope Campaigns Development Department.

Shakespeare, P., Atkinson, D. and French, S. (eds) (1993) *Reflecting on Research Practice: Issues in Health and Social Welfare*. Buckingham: Open University Press.

Shakespeare, T. (1996) Rules of engagement: doing disability research, *Disability and Society*, 11 (1): 115–19.

Shakespeare, T. (1997) ' "No choice, no voice": the exclusion of disabled children', unpublished occasional paper. University of Leeds, Disability Research Unit.

Skelton, J., Beazley, S., Maelzer, J., Moore, M. and Patient, M. (forthcoming) *Learning Disabled People and Older Care-Givers*. Disability Studies Team Project Report. Manchester: Manchester Metropolitan University.

Smith, F. (1994) *Personal Guide to The Children Act 1989 for Education Staff in England and Wales*. Sanderstead: Children Act Enterprises.

Stevenson, C. and Cooper, N. (1997) Qualitative and quantitative research, *The Psychologist*, 10 (4): 159–60.

Stokes, S. and Whitehill, T. (1996) Speech error patterns in Cantonese-speaking children with cleft palate, *European Journal of Disorders of Communication*, 31 (1): 45–64.

Stone, E. and Priestley, M. (1996) Parasites, pawns and partners: disability research and the role of non-disabled researchers, *British Journal of Sociology*, 47 (4): 609–716.

Swain, J. (1993) Taught helplessness? Or a say for disabled students in schools, in J. Swain, V. Finkelstein, S. French and M. Oliver (eds) *Disabling Barriers: Enabling Environments*. London: Sage.

Todd, S. and Shearn, J. (1997) Family dilemmas and secrets: parents' disclosure of information to their adult offspring with learning disabilities, *Disability and Society*, 12 (3): 341–66.

UNICEF (1995) *The Convention on the Rights of the Child*. London: UK Committee for UNICEF.

Webster, A. and Ellwood, J. (1985) *The Hearing-impaired Child in the Ordinary School*. London: Croom Helm.

Webster, A. and Wood, D. (1989) *Special Needs in Ordinary Schools: Children with Hearing Difficulties*. London: Cassell.

Whyte, W. F. (ed.) (1991) *Participatory Action Research*. London: Sage.

Woodford, D. (1995) Cochlear implant, in *Cochlear Implant and Bilingualism*, Kimpton: LASER.

Woolgar, S. (1988) *Science: The Very Idea*. London: Routledge.

Woolgar, S. (1993) Ethnography: a sceptical descriptive analysis of the taken-for-granted. Paper presented at Qualitative Research Methods for Psychologists Workshop. Windsor (Brunel University).

Zarb, G. (1992) On the road to Damascus: first steps towards changing the relations of disability research production, *Disability, Handicap and Society*, 7 (2): 125–38.

Zarb, G. (ed.) (1995) *Removing Disabling Barriers*. London: Policy Studies Institute.

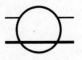

Index

STRUGGLES FOR INCLUSIVE EDUCATION
AN ETHNOGRAPHIC STUDY

Anastasia D. Vlachou

This is a lucid, authoritative and original study of teachers' views and attitudes towards the integration into mainstream schooling of a particular group of children defined as having special educational needs. It offers one of the clearest and most comprehensive analyses of the socio-political mechanisms by which the 'special' are socially constructed and excluded from the normal education system that has so far been produced.

Sally Tomlinson,
Professor of Educational Policy at Goldsmiths College,
University of London

In its detailed analysis of primary school teachers' and pupils' attitudes towards integration, this book locates the question of inclusive education within the wider educational context. The wealth of original interview material sheds new light on the reality of everyday life in an educational setting, and shows us the nature and intensity of the struggles experienced by both teachers and pupils in their efforts to promote more inclusive school practices. The author's sensitive investigation of the relationship between teachers' contradictory views of the 'special' and their integration, and the wider social structures in which teachers work, adds to our understanding of the inevitable difficulties in promoting inclusive educational practices within a system which functions via exclusive mechanisms.

The book will be of interest to students of education, sociology and disability as well as teachers and policy-makers involved in inclusive education. The original methodologies adopted when working with the children will also appeal to students of attitudinal, disability and educational research.

Contents
Introduction – Part 1: Setting the theoretical scene – Disability, normality and special needs – Towards a better understanding of attitudes – Part 2: Teachers' perspectives – Teachers and the changing culture of teaching – Teachers' attitudes towards integration (with reference to pupils with Down's Syndrome) – Part 3: Children's perspectives – Integration: the children's point of view – Disabled children and children's culture – Conclusion – Appendix 1: The problem of ethical integrity – Appendix 2: Participants in the study – Appendix 3: The role of the photograph in interviews with children – References – Index.

208 pp   0 335 19763 9 (Paperback)   0 335 19764 7 (Hardback)

DEAF AND DISABLED, OR DEAFNESS DISABLED?
TOWARDS A HUMAN RIGHTS PERSPECTIVE

Mairian Corker

Deaf people's quest for self-definition and self-determination has tended to take one of two divergent paths each embracing vastly different and often conflicting conceptualizations of deafness and disability and their relationships to contemporary socio-cultural and political contexts. Because fragmentation works against collective empowerment and effective political challenges to oppression, there is a great need to identify a common discourse which all deaf and disabled people can share without compromising fundamental beliefs and values. This book is the first to use a multi-disciplinary, postmodernist approach in the search for an inclusive framework for understanding deafness and disability, which aims to liberate the political potential of socio-cultural diversity and develop our thinking about disability as a form of social oppression. In using this approach, it exposes the essentialism inherent in existing social, political and service frameworks which confuse issues of needs and rights and contribute to the creation and reinforcement of the power imbalances at the heart of disability oppression.

Contents

176pp   0 335 19699 3 (Paperback)   0 335 19700 0 (Hardback)